DISCLAIMER:

The information that follows, including but not limited to, text, graphics, images, and other material, is for educational purposes only. The content contained within is not intended as a substitute for one-on-one professional medical advice, diagnosis, or treatment.

Always seek advice from a qualified health care provider regarding your current medical condition or treatment, and before undertaking a new health care regime.

TABLE OF CONTENTS

DEDICATION

To the still hopeful and willing

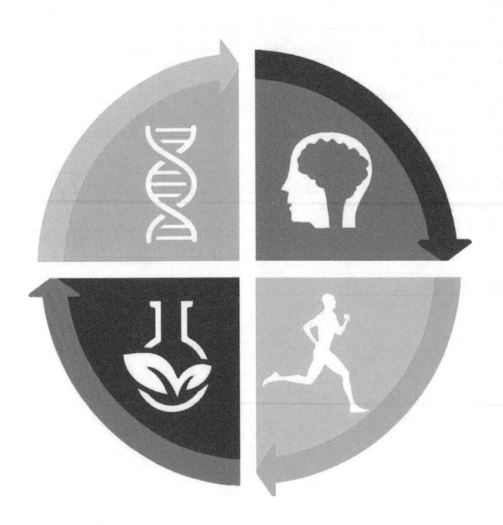

PART 1: THE CORE 4

YOU ARE NOT ALONE

The civilized world has several major health crises. The infographic from the Center for Disease Control's website shows that 6 in 10 adults have at least one well-known disease!

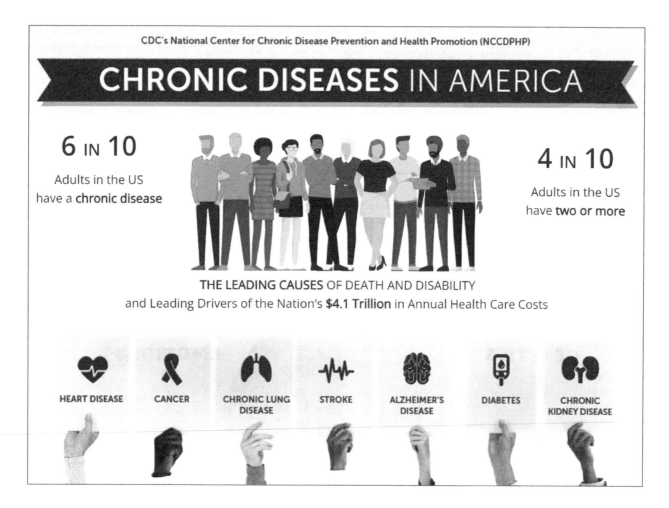

This data is shocking (and mostly preventable). But what about physical or emotional problems that are not classified as diseases such as migraines, PMS, ADHD, most pain, chronic fatigue syndrome, fibromyalgia, GERD, IBS, anxiety, insomnia, and dozens more? These ailments are called FUNCTIONAL ILLNESSES. They are often quite concerning or even scary. **In fact, nearly all non-emergency medical visits are triggered by functional illnesses.** One or more of them may be motivating you to read this book right now.

I would not be surprised to hear that in addition to your existing condition you also have doctor fatigue, diet fatigue, a shrinking bank account, and borderline hopelessness. Oh yes, you may also have a few extra symptoms and side effects from the pharmacopeia of medicines and supplements you are expected to rotate through daily. I know because I see it daily in my practice from people just like you.

You are the reason I wrote the *50 FIX Guidebook.*

WHY HASN'T MY DOCTOR BEEN ABLE TO HELP ME?

Most medical doctors are specialists in one system of the body. Specialized doctors prescribe specialized treatments. The blood test showed your hormones were off—see the endocrinologist. Your skin is dry, patchy, and inflamed—see the dermatologist. You experience heart palpitations—see the cardiologist. You suffer from an irritable bowel—see the gastroenterologist. You are anxious or depressed—see the psychiatrist. All your joints hurt—see the rheumatologist. STOP!

That has all been tried. Staying on that path means you will likely need the oncologist, anesthesiologist, and radiologist. You do not need a new specialist who will prescribe another medicine for a single problem and then send you off to a different specialist who will do the same thing. You are suffering from a whole-body wildfire that a single system treatment will never extinguish. This common oversight is due to an absence of the "big picture."

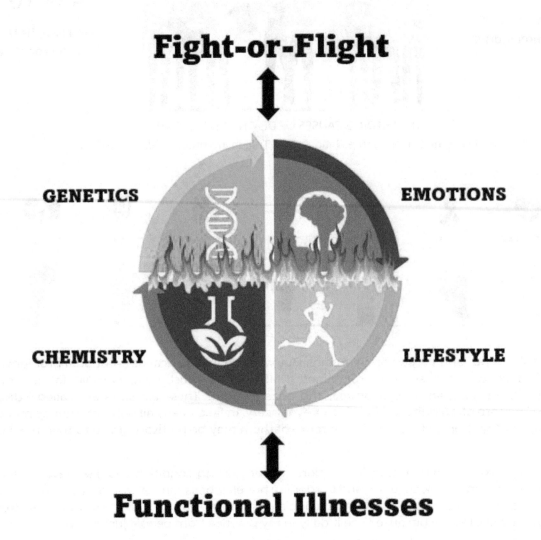

THE BIG PICTURE

The big picture is that there are four foundational requirements for health that specialists rarely discuss in conjunction. **The CORE 4 are the Genetic, Emotional, Chemical, and Lifestyle CORES.** Health is balance between them. When one CORE is off kilter, then the other three will forfeit resources attempting to buoy it. However, persistent imbalances lead to deficiencies in health-stabilizing nutrients and an erratic central nervous system. Inevitably, strong symptoms, ailments, and conditions are expressed in the form of a functional illness. But what caused the instability in the first place? To answer this question, we must understand a crucial but often unconsidered reality:

> CORE 4 imbalances either cause, or are caused by the stress response, commonly known as fight-or-flight.

There is no escaping it. Either you acquired a functional illness from long-term fight-or-flight (FOF) or some outside event (infection, toxicity, trauma, etc.) jump started a functional illness that then turned on the stress response. Either way, FOF must be regulated if health is to be achieved.

THE FIGHT-OR-FLIGHT RESPONSE

The FOF response is a physiological beast of burden, designed to use its great strength to perform important tasks of survival in times of need. It is a necessary chemical feedback loop that is meant to ramp up quickly in reaction to a threat and then return to its prior calm, fear-free state. However, if the FOF response is turned on too often the brain and central nervous system become "trained" to keep it on, or worse yet, they "forget" how to turn it off. Now the chemicals adrenaline and noradrenaline relentlessly surge throughout the body extracting massive resources from all other systems and forcing them to bend to their will, even transforming the brain itself. This is the epidemic of **ADRENALINE DOMINANCE**.

THE MANY NAMES OF FIGHT-OR-FLIGHT

The chronic state of fight-or-flight has been called by many names through the years. Since FOF is turned on automatically by the brain it is sometimes called **autonomic dysfunction or dysautonomia**. The part of the autonomic nervous system directly related to FOF is the sympathetic nervous system, so FOF is sometimes called **sympathetic overload**. All the sympathetic nerves related to the release of FOF chemicals, like adrenaline, come from nerve bundles on the front of the central thoracic spine, so FOF is sometimes called **central nervous system disorder**. To keep it simple, I associate FOF with its most famous chemical adrenaline, so I call the entire process with all its variations, **adrenaline dominance**.

THE ADRENAL GLANDS AND THEIR HORMONES

If you have been to any professional of natural health, you have likely heard about the adrenal glands or even been told you have "adrenal gland fatigue." If a functional illness has been part of your life for a few years or more, it is likely you do. These glands are the makers of adrenaline, so we need to know a bit about them.

Your body has two adrenal glands—one atop each kidney. Acting as the peacemakers of the hormonal family, the adrenal glands will exhaust all diplomatic options while attempting to maintain metabolic order. In the end, their ongoing involvement and intrusiveness irritates everybody—initiating and perpetuating vicious cycles that are destructive to the entire household as seen below in the infographic...Don't be intimidated by all the detail. Throughout the *CORE Rest Plan*, I will explain what is going on in ways that will be easy to understand.

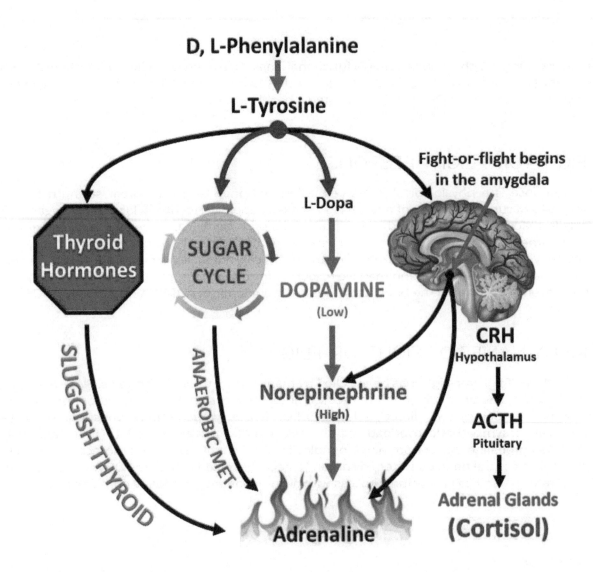

CORTISOL

Cortisol is produced in the outer part, or cortex, of the adrenal gland. It is a multi-purpose steroid hormone that has anti-viral, anti-bacterial, and anti-inflammatory properties.[1] [2] It is also a critical agent involved in blood sugar stabilization, mood balance, and restful sleep.[3] Cortisol maintains blood pressure and is important for stomach acid secretion (a very big deal I will discuss later).

EARLY-STAGE FIGHT-OR-FLIGHT (ELEVATED CORTISOL)

Chronic elevations of cortisol, like what occurs with ongoing stress, eventually suppresses the action of the immune system, thereby increasing one's chances for infection. High cortisol will also lead to weight gain by promoting fat storage and muscle tissue breakdown, a process called catabolism.[4] Two diseases relate specifically to cortisol. Cushing's syndrome is the chronic over-production of cortisol and Addison's disease is just the opposite. Both diseases are rare when compared to the functional imbalances altered adrenaline and cortisol levels create.

CORTISOL AND SLEEP

Elevated cortisol levels at night begin to disrupt sleep and make "popping out of bed" in the morning difficult. In addition, those with the profile above will likely experience sugar cravings and, if they are female, hormonal swings during their menstrual cycle.

Functional medicine doctors often make a mistake when they see this pattern by trying to force the cortisol down at night with a supplement called phosphatidyl serine. But my question is, "Why would I want to take the foot off of the brakes?" I almost never use this approach. Instead, I have opted, with much success, to take the foot off the gas pedal by calming the adrenaline response in the morning and throughout the rest of the day. This is done with the nutrients I discuss later in STEP 5 and by following the rest of the *50 FIX Plan*.

CORTISOL MAKES YOU FAT?

You may have heard that too much cortisol makes you fat. This is only partly true. Adrenaline significantly alters body metabolism to the point that you will burn up your own muscle to make sugar for your brain. Elevated levels of cortisol make this worse because of its relationship to insulin, which can promote a fat-storing process. But again, we see that adrenaline is the driving force.[5]

CORTISOL IS NOT THE STRESS HORMONE

Many healthcare professionals call cortisol the "stress hormone." I do not. ADRENALINE IS THE STRESS HORMONE. The reason cortisol got this title is because it is elevated in times of high stress. This is due to its relationship to adrenaline. Adrenaline is the gas pedal; cortisol is the brake. When stress pushes the pedal to the floor and the engine is revving at maximum RPMs, adrenaline is surging. To keep the body from going off a cliff, it must apply pressure to the brakes. Therefore, cortisol levels rapidly rise.

You can get an idea of the power of the steroid hormone cortisol by looking at synthetic prescription hormones. Cortisone, for instance, has powerful anti-inflammatory effects. MDs use cortisone to stop raging pain cycles in knees, shoulders, necks, and backs of their patients. Prednisone is used to shut down the immune system when it is causing pain, and with skin conditions like hives or eczema. Steroid inhalers are used to help people with breathing issues. Cortisol does all these things too. In fact, when someone needs these medicines for an inflammatory problem, it pretty much guarantees their cortisol levels are way too low. Some people are born with low cortisol (think children with asthma), but for most, low cortisol occurs in late-stage fight-or-flight.

LATE-STAGE FIGHT-OR-FIGHT (CORTISOL DEPLETION)

You may have heard the term, "adrenal gland exhaustion." This is not quite accurate. You have plenty of adrenaline—enough for two lifetimes. What you do not have plenty of is cortisol. So, when the adrenal glands are "exhausted" you are running on all gas pedal with no brakes. Repairing this state requires a gentle touch.

Many good doctors fail to heal their patient's adrenal glands because the supplements they use are too forceful. Most contain whole adrenal gland and high amounts of B-vitamins. Whole adrenal gland supplies the inner part, or medulla. The medulla is where adrenaline is made. We don't want any of that! Cortisol comes from our outer thin cortex. This tissue is what burns out first. So, prolonged fight-or-flight means cortisol drops dramatically.

Whole adrenal supplements do provide an energy boost, but only because they are "kicking the tired horse," forcing it to continue galloping when it is already spent. It is far too soon to rely on a supplement containing adrenal medulla. Adrenal gland restoration requires getting off the horse and walking alongside.

No matter where you are on the high or low cortisol spectrum, the processes in place are destructive in the long run and need to be addressed NOW.

YES, YOU DO HAVE FIGHT-OR-FLIGHT

Fight-or-flight often happens behind the scenes. If it happens long enough, it creates a "new normal." Most don't even realize what is happening. They will say things like, **"but I don't feel stressed."** This might be because they have adapted to their imbalances. This is quite common. Just take a look on the next page at the *50+ Ailments of Adrenaline Dominance*. These are the functional issues most people manage every day. You likely have a few or more of them too. Adding them all up it becomes more than clear that FOF overload is present.

THE 50+ AILMENTS OF ADRENALINE DOMINANCE

CENTRAL NERVOUS SYSTEM DYSREGULATION

Heart palpitations
Anxiety / Panic attacks
Numbness and tingling
Nail biting (onychophagia)
Insomnia / Restless leg syndrome
Excessive sweating (hyperhidrosis)
Cold hands and feet
Dizziness (vertigo) / POTS
Lightheadedness (usually from postural hypotension)
Shortness of breath

STOMACH SLOW DOWN

G.E.R.D. / Heartburn
Loss of appetite
Brittle or splitting nails
Excessive burping after meals
Constipation
Kidney stones
Bad breath (halitosis)

GUT INFLAMMATION

Gas / Bloating / Pain
Food sensitivities
Runny nose
Sinus Congestion / Sinusitis
Gallbladder attacks (cholecystitis)
Leaky gut syndrome
Small intestine bacterial overgrowth (SIBO)
Irritable bowel syndrome (IBS)
Yeast overgrowth (candidiasis)

BLOOD SUGAR IMBALANCES

Low blood sugar related shakiness or lightheadedness with missed meals (hypoglycemia)
Tired after eating carbohydrates - related to inadequate glucose levels inside the cells (insulin resistance)

HORMONAL DISRUPTIONS

Hormones become harder to metabolize in the liver leading to:
PMS, PCOS
Breast tenderness
Heavy bleeding, Uterine cramping
Migraine headaches
Mood disruptions (PMDD)

BRAIN STRAIN

Trouble focusing
Short-term memory loss
Poor processing of new information
Unable to turn the mind off at night
Apathy, Depression
ADHD, OCD

TOXIN ACCUMULATION

Liver sluggishness, Edema
Acne / Sensitive skin such as reactive to chemicals or jewelry
Irritability
Sensitivity to strong smells
Elevated cholesterol (hyperlipidemia)
Fatigue

MUSCULOSKELETAL DYSFUNTION

Muscle cramps and spasms
Tension headaches

IMMUNE DYSFUNCTION

Allergies to pollens or pets
Skin rashes / Hives / Eczema
Slow healing tissues
Increased susceptibility to infections and viruses

NUTRIENT DEFICIENCIES

Can lead to or perpetuate any of the 50+ ailments and promote chronic conditions like:
Fibromyalgia, Chronic fatigue syndrome

In my office I have a poster displaying the *50+ Ailments* circling the CORE 4. Hopefully this visual helps cement the idea into your mind that no system is safe from adrenaline dominance.

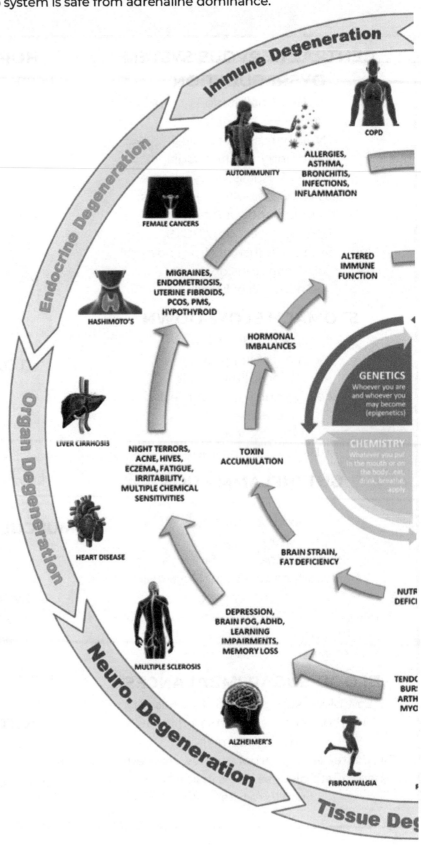

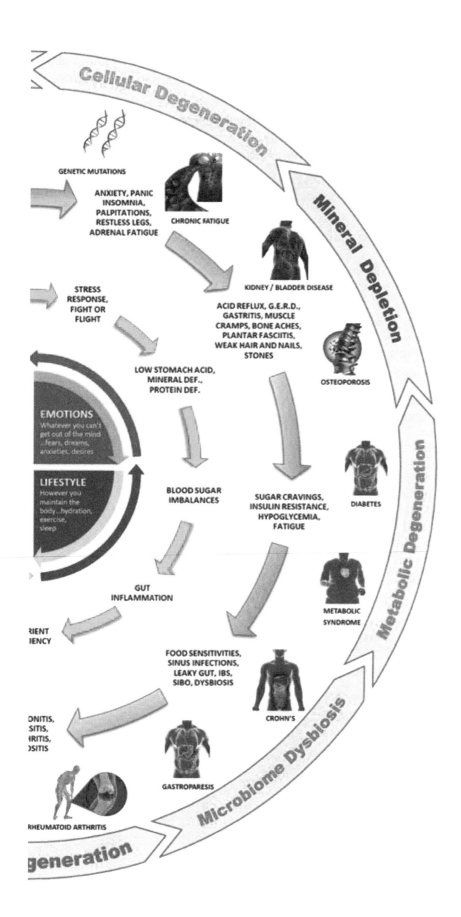

THE 10 STEPS (OVERVIEW)

After reviewing the 50+ Ailments list and my poster above you can start to see why healing adrenaline dominance by resetting the FOF response is the key to overcoming nearly all functional illnesses at the same time.

Life is an uphill journey and functional illnesses are like bricks in your backpack. The more bricks in the pack, the harder the climb. Each STEP of the *50 FIX Plan* is like removing a brick. Doing all the STEPS at the same time rebalances your CORE 4 and gives you the best chance to reach the health summit.

In my clinical practice, 85% of those who followed the 10 STEPS concurrently noticed great improvement in their symptoms including 70% of chronic sufferers with conditions other doctors could not help.

THE 10 STEPS

STEP 1: REVEAL – Stop inflammation, hormonal imbalances, and fat storage by using specific lab tests to find food allergies and nutrient deficiencies.

STEP 2: REHYDRATE – People commonly fall short in this critical component of refueling so it gets its own category. Take an inner shower by drinking ½ - 1 gallon of spring water. Also, hydrate cells and calm fight-or-flight by consuming electrolyte minerals.

STEP 3: REFUEL – For 3 to 6 weeks follow the *Gentle GI Diet* by eating three dairy-free meals per day containing protein, cooked vegetables, and a small amount of carbohydrate. Also, avoid specific raw foods, all lab created Franken-foods, and all toxic chemicals.

STEP 4: REIGNITE – Burn fat once again by waking up your sleeping metabolism.

STEP 5: REPLENISH – Experience "miracles" by using teeter-totter supplements in their proper ratios (or Core4Powder) to replenish deficient cells and tissues.

STEP 6: RESTERCISE – Exercise in your heart rate range for an optimal metabolism, not just for fitness – intense exercise increases adrenaline and trains the body to stay in fight-or-flight.

STEP 7: RESTORE – Restore sleep, balance biorhythms, and retrain the brain to relax again by following a proper nighttime routine.

STEP 8: REPLACE – Use a powerful neurological technique to remove trapped circulating emotions and replace them with calming, constructive thoughts.

STEP 9: RELOCATE – Take essential Vitamin "NO" to escape busyness, avoid high stress situations, and to prevent health setbacks.

STEP 10: RECORD – Write down your daily results and accomplishments. This keeps motivation high and maintains focus to make sure your health goals are achieved.

JUMP TO PART 4 (THE FUNCTIONAL HEALTH ASSESSMENT)

Now that you have reviewed the 10 STEPS, it is a good time to jump to the back of the *50FIX Guidebook* and complete the *Functional Health Assessment*. This will let you know just how many bricks are currently in your pack. When you are finished, return here, and keep climbing!

CORE 1: GENETICS – WHOEVER YOU ARE AND WHOEVER YOU MAY BECOME

Think of DNA as the 25,000-page blueprint for building the unique you. Each page is a gene. How well the pages are read will determine whether you are born with a deformity or later develop a disease.

For many years, scientists believed that a single bad gene was the reason for a given disease. Science now knows that a distinct gene has around 30,000 potential forms of expression.[6] This means **genes are not your destiny. They are a set of possibilities in a world of complexity.**

BILLIONS OF THEM!

If you were to see inside just one of your 100 trillion cells (yes, trillion with a "t") you would find a full copy of your 25,000-page blueprint. You would also find a factory-like world of molecular machines. There are molecular motors, propellers, switches, shuttles, nanocars, balances, tweezers, sensors, gates, assemblers, and hinges. Each cell contains billions of them!

These astoundingly complex cells are organized into tissues; tissues into organs; organs into systems; and systems into the human body. Complexity is stacked upon complexity.

All this fine-tuning keeps the body as healthy as it can be. But there are plenty of vulnerabilities. Much can and does go wrong throughout life because of *epigenetic influences.*

EPIGENETICS

The field of study known as epigenetics has taught us that external influences such as stress, poor nutrition, exercise, and even thoughts and emotions, can "program" what the gene does and when it does it. Bad influences cause "dirty genes" and result in bad outcomes, while good influences result in good outcomes.

Positive epigenetic influences are likely the reason why all women with the gene for breast cancer do not actually develop the disease. The opposite is also true.

In the womb, the behaviors of the mother regarding diet, sleep, hydration, tobacco use, alcohol consumption, etc. have a direct impact on the health of the child. If mom is toxic or immuno-compromised, then her child likely will be as well. Thankfully all is not lost.

The body is impressively resilient and operates in a non-stop state of autocorrection. Even after years of abuse or neglect, regular healthy habits and choices often lead to profound physical changes.

For example, studies of genetically identical overweight mice who came from a line of obese and immuno-compromised parents, found that their obesity could be overcome with the right nutrition. The right diet reprogrammed the genes and reshaped their genetic destiny,[7] even though the obesity was hereditary.

YOU ARE IN THE DRIVER'S SEAT!

Because the body has been designed to thrive, when you experience a functional illness like anxiety, fatigue, gut problems, headaches, etc., understand that these are flashing red lights from within signaling it is time to change course.

Every cell of your body and its DNA are now doing their part to restore balance from the inside. But the road has become too steep. They need your help! The *50 FIX Guidebook* is your map. Follow its 10 STEPS and allow their positive epigenetic influence to calm the CORE 4 from the outside.

CORE 2: EMOTIONS – WHATEVER IS IN THE MIND... FEARS, ANXIETIES, DESIRES

The powerful health disrupting effects of anxiety, fear, worry, busyness, and hopelessness are well documented. No event, past, present, or imagined in the future, occurs without an emotional component.

An otherwise strong and healthy individual who is faced with ongoing emotional distress, begins to manifest many of the signs of adrenaline dominance such as erratic moods, unstable blood sugar, adrenaline surges, disrupted sleep, drops in energy, shifts in appetite, aches, pains, and more. In other words, **they begin to express physical problems from an emotional cause.** For many, physical illness first began as an emotional imbalance.

STRESS FROM WITHOUT

Nearly one million children are victims of child abuse annually.[8] Abused and neglected children are at least 25 percent more likely than those not abused or neglected to experience problems such as delinquency, teen pregnancy, low academic achievement, drug use, and mental health problems.[9]

Abused and neglected children are 11 X more likely to be arrested for criminal behavior as juveniles, 2.7 times more likely to be arrested for violent and criminal behavior as adults, and 3.1 times more likely to be arrested for violent crimes.[10] Two-thirds of people in drug treatment programs reported being abused as children.[11]

STRESS FROM WITHIN

On the other end of the spectrum, a 2017 study on perfectionism that appeared in the journal *Psychological Bulletin* found that beginning in the 1980s, a culture of "competitive individualism" in the United States, Canada, and the United Kingdom steadily increased the quest for personal perfection.[12]

The study went on to show that current generations not only feel intense societal pressure to be perfect but also expect perfection from themselves and others. Academic performance is included in this trend, making it also a strong trigger for digestive issues from anxiety.

Young adults have always had great pressures upon them: pressures to achieve, to grow up, to be accepted, to be significant. Now, all of these are compounded by technology. Undoubtedly, these cumulative pressures, along with an open-book life on social media, are a principal reason for the shockingly high suicide rates.

STRESS OVERLOAD

The total suicide rate from 2000 to 2018 increased 30%. Suicide was the cause of 45,979 deaths in 2020. Males are four times more likely to successfully commit suicide. In the 10 to 24 age group, 81% of suicide deaths were males, 19% were females. In 2020, an estimated 12.2 million American adults seriously thought about suicide, 3.2 million planned a suicide attempt, and 1.2 million attempted suicide.

Self-harm is another direct result of emotional distress. Around 157,000 youth between the ages of 10 and 24 are treated in Emergency Departments across the U.S. for self-inflicted injuries annually.[13] **STEP 8 of the *50 FIX Plan* will teach you a powerful technique to neurologically process excess emotions.**

CORE 3: LIFESTYLE – HOWEVER YOU SLEEP OR EXERCISE

In many ways, health is like money management. First it must be earned, then wisely put to work. You might be thinking, "My body is down to its last dime." You are not alone. The entire *50 FIX Plan* is dedicated to helping you grow your health assets, while getting a return on your lifestyle investment.

Two critical lifestyle categories are proper sleep and the right form of exercise. Not sleeping is like racking up debt on your credit card for things you don't really need and having to pay the heavy interest: inflammatory reactions flare, blood sugar vacillates, and adrenaline surges. These make it much harder to get back in the black.

Not exercising is like putting money under the mattress in a time of inflation: fitness vanishes, metabolism wanes, muscles waste, and the immune system is weakened. Your overall health-value drops and what remains will not be enough when the unexpected occurs. But beware! The wrong form of exercise promotes inflammation and leads to chronic injury. In STEP 6 of the *50 FIX Plan,* I will show you how to exercise to burn fat and reduce inflammation.

MAKE LIFESTYLE HABITS

There are also no "get-rich-quick" schemes when it comes to healthy lifestyle changes. They must become habits. You will know they are habits when you crave them. Trying to get healthy by doing a thirty-day cleanse and a couch-to-10K exercise program is like trying to get an annual income with risky seasonal work. If all goes well you may catch some crabs or a boatload of fish, or you might just end up at the bottom of the Bering Sea.

This type of "getting healthy" also depends on lots of motivation and willpower, which is another big problem. Motivation is hard to maintain, and most people do not have a great deal of willpower. Only a small amount of both is required to be successful with the *50 FIX Plan.*

I highly recommend the book *Mini Habits* by Stephen Guise. It is a short read filled with lots of helpful strategies to make lifelong habits without high motivation or high willpower.

CORE 4: CHEMICAL – WHATEVER YOU EAT, DRINK, BREATHE, OR APPLY

The fourth CORE is *Chemical* and has everything to do with how well your inner nutrients are balanced. The power of proper nutrition cannot be overstated. I make a living helping patients overcome debilitating ailments using specific *hormetic* nutrients as my primary restorative therapy.

Hormesis has a Greek origin and means, "to set in motion, impel, or urge on." **A hormetic nutrient may be a single vitamin, herb or other agent that positively impacts multiple systems simultaneously.**

Any nutrient—magnesium, calcium, B vitamins, oils, antioxidants—or combinations of nutrients or botanicals (the medicines of nature) can produce a hormetic effect if they are what the body needs at that time. Utilizing these nutrients is the most efficient means of breaking disease-promoting cycles and correcting the body's chemical imbalances. Overcoming adrenaline dominance requires several hormetic nutrients. I will show you which ones they are and how they are used to balance your inner teeter-totters.

EVERYONE HAS CHEMICAL PROBLEMS

Some people think they do not have any chemical problems. However, aging itself is a chemical problem. Beyond this universal example, the person who experiences pain, insomnia, constipation, fatigue, headaches, PMS, or emotional issues such as depression or anxiety, has chemical problems. If they admit things like, "I just have a bad back (knees, hips, etc.)," or, "I get up twice a night to go to the bathroom, but that is normal," they have chemical problems. If taking over-the-counter pain, stomach, or allergy medication is a common practice, then they have chemical problems.

> In short, if the regular experience of life is anything other than a pain-free, energy-filled existence, **that person has chemical problems.**

Nothing happens in the body without countless numbers of chemical reactions taking place. There are chemical reactions that start processes and then there are other chemical reactions that stop those processes. Without the starting reaction, nothing gets going. Without the stopping reaction, everything keeps going. The chemistry necessary for starting or for stopping reactions comes from the nutrients we consume.

Just eating any food won't do—we eat plenty of food. Thirty percent of adults are obese. An additional four percent are morbidly obese. The current obesity number is double what it was just over thirty years ago.[14] The share of obese children tripled during this same time to seventeen percent.[15] And yet, nutritional deficiencies are still widespread. No, most people are not exhibiting signs of pellagra, rickets, or scurvy. But, because of their imbalanced chemistry they are experiencing a cluster of functional issues that speed them on the path of disease and prevent them from expressing optimal function.

INNER TEETER-TOTTERS

All the parts of your body are valuable, and all the parts of your body are interrelated. However, some parts are more intimately related than others through what is recognized as the *Teeter-Totter Effect.*

For example, if one nutrient is too "low," then its closely related counterpart on the other side of the teeter-totter is often too "high." Also, the more deficient or low a nutrient is, the more powerful its overall effect when *taken by itself* (full details in STEP 5).

My patients repeatedly tell me how amazed they were that their supplement program worked so fast. This is because precise replenishment of deficient nutrients produces benefits as fast-acting and powerful as pharmaceutical medicines, while balancing all teeter-totters delivers the longest lasting degree of health stability and resilience.

Some teeter-totters are not single nutrients but are instead hormones or entire systems. Here is a common listing of important teeter-totters:

- IRON, ZINC AND COPPER (A THREE-WAY TEETER-TOTTER)
- CALCIUM AND VITAMIN D AND MAGNESIUM
- VITAMINS B1 AND B2
- POTASSIUM AND SODIUM
- ADRENALINE AND CORTISOL (THE ANXIETY CHEMICALS)
- SEROTONIN AND DOPAMINE
- ESTROGEN AND PROGESTERONE
- THE IMMUNE SYSTEM (TH-1 VS. TH-2)
- THE NERVOUS SYSTEM (SYMPATHETIC VS. PARASYMPATHETIC)

When symptoms of any kind are present it is likely that a teeter-totter is broken. Migraine headaches, for example, are most often a sign of too much serotonin in the brain. However, "too much" is relative to dopamine. Therefore, a person suffering from migraines could have high serotonin with normal dopamine levels. Or, she could have normal serotonin with low dopamine levels. Either way, the teeter-totter looks the same, and the migraine symptoms are the same. However, in one case the goal is to lower serotonin, while in the other case, the goal is to raise dopamine (sometimes a person will need both).

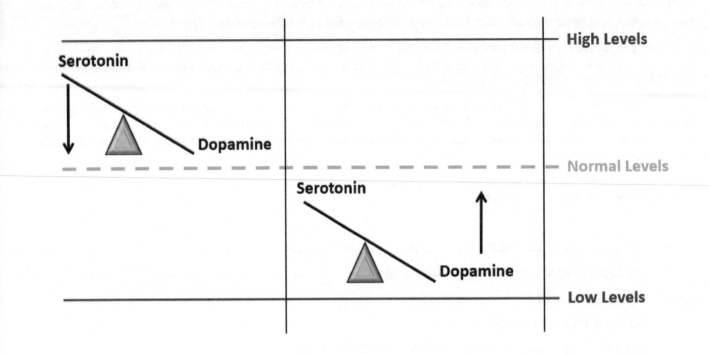

GAS PEDALS AND BRAKES

Teeter-totters could also be likened to a gas pedal and a brake. There are a set of chemicals or electrical signals that initiate the function and an opposite set of signals that suppress that same function. This balancing act is called a negative feedback loop. This loop makes sure your body does not go too fast or too slow as it tries to maintain its balance, or homeostasis.

A good example is what happens when you have a sugary drink. In the body, the sugar is turned into glucose, which rises sharply in the blood—this is the gas pedal. Extra glucose in the cells gives us energy, but elevated levels for too long are inflammatory to certain tissues—you are now going too fast. The body responds by releasing as much insulin as required (the brake) to transport the excess glucose into the cells so that the overall blood glucose level comes into balance.

PART 2: THE 50 FIX PLAN

It's time. The only way many of you reading this book can recover your health is to shut off adrenaline dominance. To do this, you must follow ALL the 10 STEPS for many WEEKS OR MONTHS.

Gone are the days when you could just hit the gym and cut back on the carbs to "lose weight and feel great." No pain, no gain no longer works. In fact, it will make things worse (see STEP 6). Only having a "little bite" of your favorite poison could be enough to ruin what you started for days at a time. No more cheating.

The good news is I have seen this program work ~~hundreds of~~ thousands of times. The STEPS are simple and do-able. But your body will resist. So, determine to get through the first week and then the weeks that follow will not be so bad. Your body will crave its new diet and lifestyle.

I guarantee, after a week or two if you have a "cheat" meal or treat you will experience a strong negative signal. Congratulations! Your body is accepting the new and rejecting the old. You are transforming your inner chemistry. You are subduing adrenaline dominance. Health is just an established routine away. Now let's get started!

THE 10 STEPS

STEP 1: REVEAL – Stop inflammation, hormonal imbalances, and fat storage by using specific lab tests to find food allergies and nutrient deficiencies.

STEP 2: REHYDRATE – People commonly fall short in this critical component of refueling so it gets its own category. Take an inner shower by drinking ½ - 1 gallon of spring water. Also, hydrate cells and calm fight-or-flight by consuming electrolyte minerals.

STEP 3: REFUEL – For 3 to 6 weeks follow the *Gentle GI Diet* by eating three dairy-free meals per day containing protein, cooked vegetables, and a small amount of carbohydrate. Also, avoid specific raw foods, all lab created Franken-foods, and all toxic chemicals.

STEP 4: REIGNITE – Burn fat once again by waking up your sleeping metabolism.

STEP 5: REPLENISH – Experience "miracles" by using teeter-totter supplements in their proper ratios (or Core4Powder) to replenish deficient cells and tissues.

STEP 6: RESTERCISE – Exercise in your heart rate range for an optimal metabolism, not just for fitness – intense exercise increases adrenaline and trains the body to stay in fight-or-flight.

STEP 7: RESTORE – Restore sleep, balance biorhythms, and retrain the brain to relax again by following a proper nighttime routine.

STEP 8: REPLACE – Use a powerful neurological technique to remove trapped circulating emotions and replace them with calming, constructive thoughts.

STEP 9: RELOCATE – Take essential Vitamin "NO" to escape busyness, avoid high stress situations, and to prevent health setbacks.

STEP 10: RECORD – Write down your daily results and accomplishments. This keeps motivation high and maintains focus to make sure your health goals are achieved.

STEP 1: REVEAL

STOP INFLAMMATION, HORMONAL IMBALANCES, AND FAT STORAGE BY USING SPECIFIC LAB TESTS TO FIND HIDDEN FOOD ALLERGIES AND NUTRIENT DEFICIENCIES

SNEAKY FOODS

There is no perfect food. All foods are guilty until proven innocent. All foods require digestion, assimilation, and elimination. Some foods are easier to process than others. But know this, there are ALWAYS a group of sneaky foods causing us harm that we do not suspect.

Every new patient in my office is asked to provide a detailed list of their regular foods. Whatever foods they eat daily are the ones I am most suspicious of. Why? Because fight-or-flight irritates the immune system. And an activated immune system is indiscriminate and will start to "tag" common foods as foreign invaders.

I also ask patients what foods they "love?" An emotional attachment to food is a clue that a chemical addiction may be present. The chemistry of addiction leads to neurological changes in the brain and causes us to crave things that are harmful to us. We need to know which foods they are. So, instead of doing an exhaustive elimination diet that could take many months, we are going to test and find out.

WHY LAB TESTING?

Some things just cannot be known without testing. Some things we never want to guess. Since our goal is to shut down adrenaline dominance, which affects EVERY system of the body, the more data the better. The number and type of possible lab tests is dizzying. Thankfully, all you need is two (maybe three) tests for these four reasons:

1. To avoid **FOOD SENSITIVITIES** – Food allergies and sensitivities cause the immune system to work overtime resulting in whole-body inflammation (think painful joints and muscles, trouble losing weight, and water retention). They are also the #1 reason adrenaline dominance is turned on in the first place.

2. To replenish **NUTRITIONAL DEFICIENCIES** – We need to know which vitamins and minerals are required to calm the CORE 4 and overcome adrenaline dominance. These are your teeter-totter nutrients as explained fully in STEP 5 (**nutritional deficiencies and chemical toxicities are combined in one lab test**).

3. To cleanse **CHEMICAL TOXICITIES** – The solution to pollution is dilution. What can't be eliminated gets stored. Adrenaline dominance stresses out the liver, colon, and kidneys making detoxification inefficient. The result is tissues full of toxins (i.e., heavy metals and metabolic waste products). The body will intentionally hold on to excess water and slow down metabolism to dilute their poisonous effects.

4. To balance **HORMONAL IRREGULARITIES** – Adrenaline dominance greatly disrupts the hormonal (endocrine) system. No hormone producing glands escape. Hypothyroidism, insulin resistance, PMS, PCOS, and infertility are just some of its effects (**this test is optional for some patients**).

LAB TEST #1 THE FOOD SENSITIVITY TEST

Here is a sample food allergy test. It measures the total amount of immunoglobulin G (IgG) created by your immune system because of specific noxious (antigenic) foods. Unlike IgE reactions that can cause immediate life-threatening anaphylaxis, IgG reactions take hours or even days to manifest their unpleasant effects. That is why we need to test them.

HOW LONG MUST I AVOID THESE FOODS?

This is not a one-and-done test. It is a snapshot telling you which foods are disruptive today. With the *50 Fix Plan* your body will be changing, healing, adapting, and regenerating. **Be sure to avoid the foods in zones I and II for 1-2 months and foods in zones III and IV for 2-4 months.** Then retest to see how much healing has taken place.

96 General Food Panel: IgG
Complete Report

Provider: Scott Monk, D.C.
Patient: Sample
Accession #: 2023004753
Collected: 2023-01-10

Sex: M
Age: 52
Received: 2023-01-20

Sample Type: DBS
Date of Birth: 1980-09-17
Completed: 2023-01-25

IgG

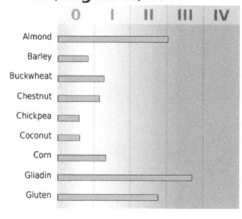

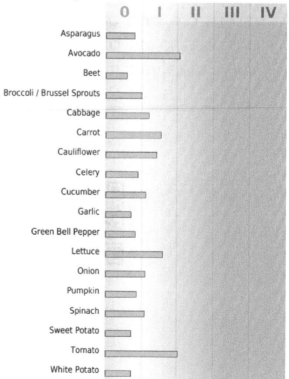

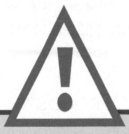

ATTENTION!

You will see a *Master Food List* in the pages ahead. This is your menu minus any foods that show reactive on your *Food Sensitivity Test*.

You will notice our *Master Food List* is a HEALTHY food list to follow. But becomes even HEALTHIER for you based on your test results.

IMPORTANT: Just because you did NOT react to wheat, barley, rye, and oats (i.e., gluten) does NOT give you a free pass to eat pizza every meal! Be sure to follow the food guidelines in STEP 3.

ORDER YOUR LABS

LAB TEST #2 THE MINERAL, VITAMIN, & HEAVY METAL REPORT

A common question that comes up is "What supplements should I be taking?" The truth is you are NOT what you eat...you are what you ABSORB. So, our answer is, let's test to find out. The most expensive vitamin is the one you don't need. So many people are taking so many things. But the question is, do they really need them?

Another common question is, "Can't I just take a good quality multivitamin?" Multivitamins are going to provide moderate amounts of everything. However, it will rarely fix a nutrient deficiency because it does not balance the body's Teeter-Totters. This is a big deal and is the reason it has its own chapter (see STEP 5).

The wise approach is nutrient testing. Don't guess...test! Doing so means you will have an objective look at exactly what vitamins / supplements need to be taken to achieve a more optimal state of health. Test to find your unique needs, then supplement to fill in the missing teeter-totter nutrients.

After a few months, retest to make sure the deficiency was corrected.

Mineral Test Report

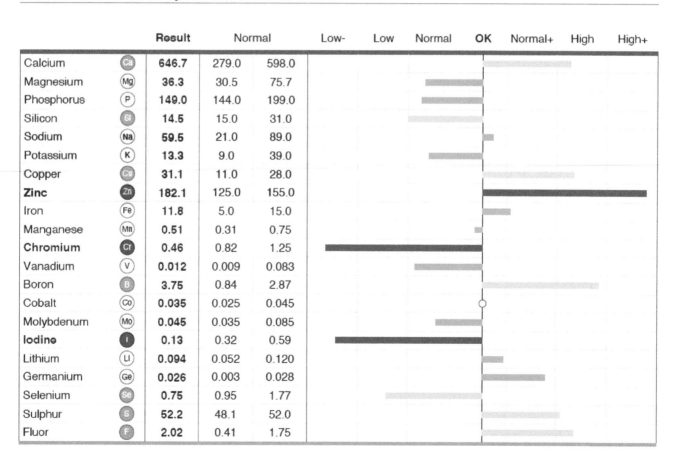

		Result	Normal		Low-	Low	Normal	OK	Normal+	High	High+
Calcium	Ca	646.7	279.0	598.0							
Magnesium	Mg	36.3	30.5	75.7							
Phosphorus	P	149.0	144.0	199.0							
Silicon	Si	14.5	15.0	31.0							
Sodium	Na	59.5	21.0	89.0							
Potassium	K	13.3	9.0	39.0							
Copper	Cu	31.1	11.0	28.0							
Zinc	Zn	182.1	125.0	155.0							
Iron	Fe	11.8	5.0	15.0							
Manganese	Mn	0.51	0.31	0.75							
Chromium	Cr	0.46	0.82	1.25							
Vanadium	V	0.012	0.009	0.083							
Boron	B	3.75	0.84	2.87							
Cobalt	Co	0.035	0.025	0.045							
Molybdenum	Mo	0.045	0.035	0.085							
Iodine	I	0.13	0.32	0.59							
Lithium	Li	0.094	0.052	0.120							
Germanium	Ge	0.026	0.003	0.028							
Selenium	Se	0.75	0.95	1.77							
Sulphur	S	52.2	48.1	52.0							
Fluor	F	2.02	0.41	1.75							

Vitamins

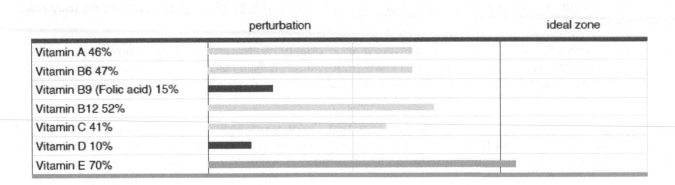

	perturbation	ideal zone
Vitamin A 46%		
Vitamin B6 47%		
Vitamin B9 (Folic acid) 15%		
Vitamin B12 52%		
Vitamin C 41%		
Vitamin D 10%		
Vitamin E 70%		

Heavy Metal Test Report

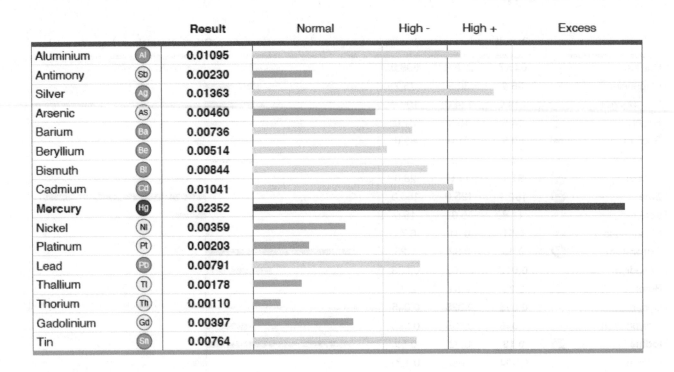

		Result	Normal	High -	High +	Excess
Aluminium	Al	0.01095				
Antimony	Sb	0.00230				
Silver	Ag	0.01363				
Arsenic	As	0.00460				
Barium	Ba	0.00736				
Beryllium	Be	0.00514				
Bismuth	Bi	0.00844				
Cadmium	Cd	0.01041				
Mercury	Hg	0.02352				
Nickel	Ni	0.00359				
Platinum	Pt	0.00203				
Lead	Pb	0.00791				
Thallium	Tl	0.00178				
Thorium	Th	0.00110				
Gadolinium	Gd	0.00397				
Tin	Sn	0.00764				

THE ORIGIN OF FOOD INTOLERANCES AND NUTRIENT DEFICIENCIES?

The Industrial Revolution led to the introduction of sucrose (white sugar), mass-produced meats, refined grains, refined vegetable oils, hydrogenated oils, and high fructose corn syrup (HFCS). It also created ways of extracting oils and nutrients from foods to extend the shelf-life, which made it possible to transport them across great distances without spoilage. However, what was good for convenience and mass consumption was not necessarily good for physiology. The refining processes greatly diminished, or stripped out completely, the natural essential nutrients and replaced them with synthetic versions.

Worse yet, many foods are also genetically modified (GM or GMO). The modifications do cause greater yields, help plants resist bugs, and protect food from potent insecticides and herbicides. Unfortunately, unlike the selective breeding and farming done since the beginning to encourage desirable traits, scientists are tinkering with the genetic code of foods with some very unpleasant results. Instead of using nature to bring about the healthiest and most productive crops, they have created a world of Franken-foods, the effects of which are not fully known.

Researchers may take pride in creating a chemical-resistant food crop that when sprayed with insecticides and herbicides will kill everything in the field except the plant itself. However, common sense screams that serving Franken-foods for dinner is a recipe for monsters and nightmares. In my experience, a primary reason for food allergies and consequent nutrient deficiencies is overconsumption of manipulated foods.

POOR ABSORPTION

With digestive challenges such as leaky gut, celiac disease, Crohn's disease, IBS etc. on the rise...the cascade effect is poor absorption or malabsorption of key nutrients and vitamins necessary for optimal health and function.

Another important concept to understand is this: roughly 40% of the U.S. is "sensitive" to gluten, meaning it irritates the small intestine, the place where most nutrient absorption occurs. True gluten allergies literally carve off the absorbing villi creating inflammation and an erratic, overactive immune system.

Gluten sensitivity, or any food intolerance for that matter, guarantees nutrient deficiencies through poor absorption. It is simply harder to get the necessary nutrients into the bloodstream and into the cells.

PRESCRIPTION MEDICATIONS

This list could go on for a hundred pages. Simply put, EVERY medication drains the body of certain nutrients. This is no surprise because every type of stress does the same thing. Here are a few examples:

NSAIDS (Motrin, Aleve, Advil etc.) can lead to deficiencies of folic acid (vitamin B9), pantothenic acid (vitamin B5), vitamin C, and Iron.

Anti-inflammatories like prednisone can lead to deficiencies in vitamin D, vitamin C, vitamin B6, vitamin B12 and vitamin B9 (folic acid).

Meanwhile statin drugs prescribed to reduce cholesterol, drain the cells of the energy making CO-Q-10.

Acid blockers, one of the most used OTC medications, greatly reduce hydrochloric acid (HCl) in the stomach which guarantees poor protein digestion and mineral absorption since both are HCl dependent.

STEP 2: REHYDRATE

TAKE AN INNER SHOWER BY DRINKING ½ - 1 GALLON OF SPRING WATER. ALSO HYDRATE CELLS AND CALM FIGHT-OR-FLIGHT BY CONSUMING ELECTROLYTE MINERALS

Electrolytes are one of the safest and fastest ways to calm anxiety. The reason is electrolytes are the first set of nutrients to be depleted when the body is under the influence of adrenaline dominance. These are the same nutrients lost through sweat during heat exposure, exercise, or athletics. In the extreme, these three situations can also further encourage fight-or-flight creating a viscous cycle.

WHAT ARE ELECTROLYTES?

In nutrition, "electrolyte" refers to essential minerals found in your blood, sweat and urine that carry a positive or negative electric charge. Electrolytes play a vital role in nerve impulse conduction, muscle contraction, muscle relaxation, cellular hydration, and regulation of the body's internal pH levels. Common electrolytes found in your body include:

- Sodium
- Potassium
- Chloride
- Calcium
- Magnesium
- Phosphate
- Bicarbonate

In the stomach under the influence of high amounts of acid, these minerals are broken down, or metabolized, forming electrolytes with positively or negatively charged elements (ions).

BLOOD TESTS OFTEN MISS CELLULAR DEHYDRATION

People with adrenaline dominance often have significant nutritional deficiencies within their cells despite a standard blood test showing the sodium, calcium, and potassium levels within a normal range. This is because the body's highest priority is to have its blood contents maintained in balanced and with adequate quantities. This means cells will become "dehydrated" by offering up any excess intracellular nutrients for the benefit of the blood. These sacrifices are necessary but exact a substantial health toll. Consuming regular doses of electrolytes is the fastest way to replenish depleted cells and restore the body's fluid balance.

ELECTROLYTE IMBALANCES

Electrolyte imbalances are the hallmark of prolonged fight-or-flight and are the source of many functional illnesses. The symptoms of electrolyte deficiency generally happen gradually over time. However, in cases such as excessive heat, extreme exertion, vomiting or diarrhea they can happen rapidly within hours or minutes and include:

- Fatigue
- Fast or irregular heartbeat
- Numbness and tingling
- Muscle cramping / weakness
- Headaches
- Confusion
- Convulsions

MY STORY

My personal experience with electrolyte depletion and its scary signs was the reason I became interested in the natural health field. In college I was a member of the University of Florida baseball team. Most days consisted of two and a half hours of practice under the Florida sun. You can imagine my regular appearance: a fully drenched uniform and skin striped with a farmer's tan. The soaked zebra look was humorous on the outside, but something serious was taking place on the inside. A white salt-stained ring around the base of my ball cap was a sure sign I was losing electrolytes...lots of them.

The gradual loss of these critical minerals took a toll on my physiology. For many nights in a row when I would lie down to sleep, my heart would begin to speed up, slow down, and skip beats. Was I having a heart attack? Was something seriously wrong with me? Uncertainty created its own emotional anxiety, making the problem worse. The frightening symptoms would come and go over the next year, ranging from mild and hardly noticeable to severe at times, seemingly without any connection to my lifestyle.

It turned out I just needed a simple potassium supplement. Within a week all my symptoms vanished and did not return. That was the first time I saw the power of proper nutrition. Now I see it every day with my patients. If you follow the 10 STEPS of the *50 FIX Plan,* I expect you will experience it too.

HOMEMADE ELECTROLYTE DRINK

There are plenty of good electrolyte products on the market these days—especially my customized product, *Core4Powder* (discussed in STEP 5). If you choose one of them, make sure it has at least 300mg of potassium and 150mg of sodium. Also make sure that these are not carbonate forms. Carbonate (or bicarbonate) is extremely alkalizing. And as you learn in STEP 3, acidifying the stomach and digestive tract is the key to mineral absorption and protein digestion. So, we do not want to sabotage this process by using alkalizing substances (I know, many of you have been led to believe you should be following an alkalizing diet. I detail why THIS IS NOT A GOOD IDEA in PART 3: *Alkaline Water and Alkaline Food Myths*).

Making an electrolyte drink at home is quite easy. Here are the basics:

- Sea salt (1/4 tsp) in 12 ounces of water

- Potassium citrate (1/2 tsp) or coconut water (12 ounces)

- Honey or cane sugar (1 tsp) — these aid in mineral absorption. *No additional sugar is necessary in sweetened coconut water.*

- Optionally add lime, ginger and/or herbal tea for flavor.

- Sip up to 24 ounces-worth throughout the day.

- Additionally, remember to drink at least one half of your body weight in ounces of filtered or spring water per day.

STEP 3: REFUEL WITH THE GENTLE GI OR GENTLE AI DIET

EAT 3 DAIRY-FREE MEALS PER DAY THAT CONTAIN PROTEIN, COOKED VEGETABLES, AND A SMALL AMOUNT OF CARBOHYDRATE, WHILE AVOIDING ALL RAW OR ABRASIVE FOODS

Your goal is not a fad diet, but a lifestyle diet. To get there, we always start with the *Gentle GI Diet* with or without snacks. The snacks will help stabilize blood sugar swings. This is critical for those of you with hypoglycemia. Eventually, the snacks can be dropped and if you are trying to lose weight, the carbs are also dropped to as low as **50 GRAMS** per day if necessary, depending upon your glucose levels (discussed in STEP 4). Besides snacks, if you have certain chronic issues or autoimmune disease, you should begin the more restrictive *Gentle AI Diet.*

GENTLE GI DIET

The *Gentle GI Diet* prioritizes the elimination of milk-products from animals above other foods since milk-products are the most common irritant to the linings of the stomach and gut. This constant irritation promotes inflammation and immune system overactivation since 60% of the immune system is in the gut lining. Over time, more foods and food ingredients like gluten that were once manageable for many, become targets of the hyperactive immune system. Ultimately food sensitivities and food allergies result. Thankfully, many who thought they had a gluten allergy can once again eat gluten after healing their gut with the *Gentle GI Diet.* Others, however, need an even stronger diet to reset their CORE.

GENTLE AI DIET

The *Gentle AI Diet* is for those who have true gluten sensitivity, celiac disease, autoimmunity, or other inflammatory conditions (see examples below). If that is you, your dietary choices will be significantly reduced. This is non-negotiable. It will be necessary to avoid animal milk products, gluten, eggs, corn, soy, peanuts and more to feel well and balanced. Don't worry. You can do it. I give you a *Master Food List* and a clear path to follow. Just read all the details of the *Gentle GI Diet* in this chapter so that you understand the principles. Then see the *Gentle AI Diet* for the extra exemptions and exclusions.

Autoimmune Diseases

- Hashimoto's
- Rheumatoid arthritis
- Lupus
- Celiac disease
- Sjogren's syndrome
- Polymyalgia rheumatica
- Multiple sclerosis
- Type 1 diabetes
- Psoriasis

Chronic Illnesses

- Fibromyalgia
- S.E.I.D. - Systemic Exertion Intolerance Disease (chronic fatigue syndrome)
- Multiple chemical sensitivities (MCS)
- Lyme's disease
- Crohn's disease
- Type 2 diabetes
- Eczema

GENTLE GI DIET

The *Gentle GI Diet* is designed for the majority of people. Its purpose is to correct several of the systems influenced by adrenaline dominance at the same time. The *Gentle GI Diet* promotes the use of soft, well-cooked foods to allow the underperforming stomach and its irritated lining to heal, and then, by extension, the rest of the gut as well. Meanwhile, the protein eaten at each meal regulates blood sugar swings and their consequent hormonal imbalances. All these positive changes promote an easy and natural detoxification, taking the strain off the liver and kidneys, while greatly reducing whole-body inflammation.

EXAMPLE FOODS

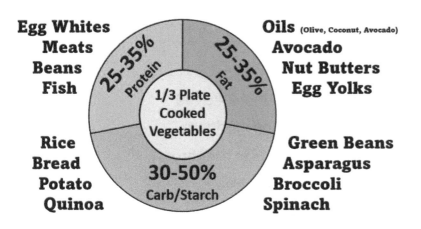

HOW LONG?

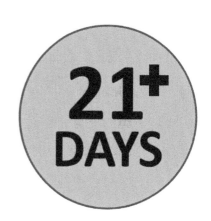

WHEN TO EAT? – WITHIN 40 MINUTES

BUT I AM NOT HUNGRY WHEN I WAKE UP?

That is not surprising. All night long your body has been managing the adrenaline surges that began from gradually dropping blood sugar levels. These surges, on top of the ones you are already experiencing from imbalances in the CORE 4, mean that you have been in fight-or-flight all night long while trying to sleep and heal. It likely meant that you were **catabolic - breaking down your own muscle to make sugar (glucose) for your brain.** This cycle must be broken.

You can stop this by having a protein/fat/carbohydrate breakfast within **the first 40 minutes** of being awake. If in the first few days you cannot tolerate a full meal, have half, or a third of a meal. Forcing your body to eat in the morning is training. Your body will do what you train it to do. Eating in the morning will raise blood sugar levels to normal. This calms adrenaline surges and halts the muscle-wasting, fat-storing catabolic process.

ALWAYS "LISTEN" TO YOUR BODY

You are about to make big beneficial changes to your diet. But everything may not go smoothly. So, pay attention to what your body has to "say."

Our bodies are always talking. How we feel – tired/energetic, motivated/apathetic, pain-free/achy - are all "conversations" your body is having with your mind. So, we need to listen.

Listening to your body simply means becoming aware of any changes that occur after drinking or eating. Negative signals indicate that a food has become hurtful, not helpful. It is not uncommon for foods, even "healthy" foods, to cause problems in different people. It is important therefore, to discern between those foods that react well with your body and those that do not.

The technique is simple. Think about how your body feels before you eat. After you have eaten and within the next hour or so, analyze yourself again. Do you now experience any symptoms? Did the ones you already had get any worse? If so, you can be sure that your body has a problem with one or more of the foods you just ate.

- Bloating
- Burping
- Dizziness
- Fatigue / sleepiness
- Gas
- Headache
- Increased heart rate

- Intestinal gurgling
- Lightheadedness
- Mucous in the throat
- Stiff muscles
- Stuffiness in the head or sinuses
- Tight joints
- Weakness

This technique will get easier the longer you eat healthfully. Practice is also important. The more you practice this technique, the easier it is to "hear" the right information.

ADD SOME FIBER

For a few, the most common issue when switching to the *Gentle GI Diet* is constipation. Because the *Gentle GI Diet* takes away the "roughage" of raw foods to allow the stomach to heal, it is missing some of the fiber necessary for proper motility. Therefore, adding fiber in the short-term may be required.

Fibers come in two types: soluble and insoluble. Insoluble fibers positively affect elimination by promoting increased peristalsis (wave-like motion of intestines) and bulking effects. Soluble fibers promote cardiovascular health, help maintain cholesterol levels, and promote the growth of good bacteria. **Look for products that contain chia seed or flaxseed, orange pulp & peel, and/or apple pectin.**

DO A 75% GENTLE GI DIET IF NECESSARY

If, after adding in daily fiber some constipation remains, then modify the *Gentle GI Diet* slightly by adding in additional fruit or a salad every other day. Stick mostly to mixed greens, carrot slices and pealed cucumber while keeping seeds at a minimum and using a low-sugar dressing.

WHAT TO EAT? – EAT SOFT FOODS (NOTHING RAW)

A stomach compromised from fight-or-flight has been "sprained" and needs to be taken out of the game, placed on injured reserve, and given little work to do while it heals. This "resting phase" occurs by only providing mostly broken down—well cooked—foods. Foods in this state can quickly be moved through the stomach and into the small intestine for further digestion. Raw foods are to be avoided because they are abrasive to the already irritated stomach lining.

Near the end of this chapter, you will find your Master Food List. Use this list for your grocery shopping and meal preparation. Below, I explain why you will be eating these selected foods.

EAT HIGH QUALITY PROTEIN ALL MEALS

Protein has many benefits including:

1. Stabilizing blood sugar swings by modulating the amount of insulin secreted by the pancreas.

2. Reducing adrenaline levels and the muscle wasting that comes with chronically high adrenaline.

3. Providing the necessary amino acids for muscle repair and brain hormones (neurotransmitters).

4. Stimulating acid production in the stomach.

5. Transforming a yeast-filled microbiome into a more balanced and healthy gut flora.

WATCH OUT FOR CHEMICALS —Be sure to greatly minimize processed meats that contain antibiotics, MSG, hormones, nitrates, nitrites, chemical preservatives, and artificial flavors or colors.

All these benefits are predicated on the necessity of proper acid levels in the stomach, which is why an acid supplement is almost always a must as discussed in *STEP 5: Replenish your Teeter-Totters.*

EAT PLENTY OF COOKED VEGETABLES AND SOME SIMPLE CARBS

We need the fiber, vitamins, and minerals from vegetables. Yes, many nutrients will be lost due to cooking. That is okay, you will catch up on food-based nutrition later. First, the gut must be healed. So, aim for 1/3 to 1/2 a plate of cooked vegetables. Carbohydrates like rice, potato, corn, and wheat can be part of your 1/4 plate of carbs.

FERMENTED FOODS

SAUERKRAUT OR KIMCHI (non-spicy) — Eat 1/4 cup every other day of these fermented foods. They are both naturally full of beneficial bacteria and gut healing properties. Sauerkraut contains high levels of glutamic acid and folic acid. These are excellent tissue-healing agents, especially in the gut.

EAT HIGH QUALITY FATS

Fats make up 50% of the brain and are foundational for cell membranes and nerve coatings. Fats are greatly beneficial for controlling inflammation, hormonal balance, cellular detoxification, and brain neurotransmission. In your diet, be sure to include plenty of organic and cold-pressed oils, such as olive oil, avocado oil, and coconut oil. Also, eat avocados, eggs, nut butters, high quality meats, salmon, and organic grass-fed butter.

BEVERAGES

DRINK ½ YOUR BODY WEIGHT IN OUNCES OF WATER PER DAY — Noncaffeinated teas, or herbal tea are also acceptable. If they are lightly sweetened, then only drink them with a protein meal or snack.

REDUCE CAFFEINATED BEVERAGES — If you "can't live without my coffee," this proves you are operating in a state of adrenaline dominance and are relying on adrenaline surges to provide you with low-quality energy just to get going. Cut your caffeine intake in half right away as you work toward zero caffeine within the first two weeks.

COFFEE CREAMER – The non-dairy, plant-based, or nut-based forms do not usually contain any alkalizing calcium carbonate and so may be used. Do not consume more than one ounce per cup.

LITTLE OR NO ALCOHOL – Many patients fail to get well because they enjoy a glass of wine every night. Beer and wine are fermented and promote yeast growth and frequently tax the liver. An overworked liver can lead to trouble falling asleep, restless sleep throughout the night, and hormonal stress. Have no alcohol for the first two weeks. If resuming alcohol after that time causes sleep to become disrupted, then eliminate alcohol entirely.

SUGARS

Sugar can be used to help calm the fight-or-flight response if consumed wisely. However, most people overdo it. A barely sweetened cup of noncaffeinated tea is helpful in the morning if breakfast is within 20 minutes.

NEVER eat sweet foods by themselves, especially before bed. There must always be protein present, otherwise, the body will be forced to produce insulin and adrenaline surges to manage the glucose. If this happens the entire insulin/cortisol/adrenaline cascade is ignited, and major setbacks occur.

> **NO SUGARS** – Do not eat any sweets if you have signs of yeast overgrowth (bloating after carbohydrates, vaginal itching, anal itching, or recent nail fungus) or if you have insulin resistance (tired after meals or loss of brain focus after meals). In the future, when your CORE 4 has improved, you may have a small amount of a sweet.

> **CAN I EAT FRUIT?** – Yes, but always with protein. With larger fruits like apples, pears, peaches, etc., have them skinless for the first 3 weeks. Limit your fruit to one small serving every other day.

> **ARTIFICIAL SWEETENERS?** – Avoid all artificial sweeteners.

> **NATURAL SWEETENERS?** – Stevia, erythritol, or monk fruit are acceptable every other day. Be sure to rotate between the various ones. For some people, honey is not a problem, for some it is. Start with none. As you improve in the weeks ahead, you can have a small amount.

> **CONDIMENTS?** – Avoid sugar-filled condiments such as ketchup. Mustard and mayonnaise are acceptable.

EAT A PROTEIN SNACK

Blood sugar spikes and dips are one of the fastest ways to turn on fight-or-flight and get stuck in adrenaline dominance. I teach you how to figure out your unique blood sugar swings in STEP 4. If you become shaky, lightheaded, or "hangry" with missed or delayed meals (hypoglycemia), you need snacks.

Some say they do not experience these symptoms but be sure that blood sugar issues are ALWAYS present with anxiety, cold hands and feet, excessive sweating, hormonal imbalances, sleep issues and more. If this describes you, a protein/fat/lower carb snack between meals we be critical.

Once blood sugar is greatly stabilized, the snacks can be dropped and periods without food can be used for weight loss purposes. How long you go without food will be determined by your blood sugar levels (STEP 4).

WHAT ABOUT SOY PROTEIN?

Soy increases estrogen and makes it more difficult for estrogen to be metabolized in the liver. So, no soy for boy! Likewise, menstruating women with ANY hormonal or PMS issues at all, should not use soy products.

PRE-MADE SNACK EXAMPLES

EGG MUFFINS	Bake scrambled eggs mixed with cooked vegetables and a small amount of rice or potato in a muffin pan sprayed with olive oil
CHICKEN OR TUNA SALAD	You can have a spoonful or two of this along with a couple bites of carrot or a few berries
NUT BUTTER WITH APPLE OR CELERY	Remove the skin on the apples for the first three weeks
MEAT JERKY	Can be eaten with a few bites of rice or potato
HUMMUS AND VEGGIES	Can be eaten with a few rice crackers
DELI MEAT ROLL UPS	Use high-quality, no added chemical lunch meat. This can also be eaten with a bite or two of carbs
PROTEIN OR BONE BROTH SHAKE (1 CUP)	Make sure it is non-soy, non-whey, and non-chocolate flavored
LEFTOVERS	Have a bite or two of your leftover meat and vegetable dinner

WHAT TO AVOID (DAIRY, CHOCOLATE, POPCORN, ETC.)

EMOTIONAL FOODS LIE

"But I love chocolate (wine, milk, cheese, etc.)." Most people do. After you have healed your gut with the *Gentle GI Diet* and calmed the rest of the CORE 4, it may be that you can enjoy them in moderation from time to time.

Eat to live. Do not live to eat. Eating and drinking daily only what you love is a near guarantee of addictive chemistry and the inflammatory effects it brings. The worse off you are, the more strictly you must avoid things that are harmful. Be highly suspicious of emotional foods and avoid them. It is always best to save emotional foods for times of celebration.

MILK-BASED PRODUCTS

Do not consume milk even if you do not have an allergy. The carbonate/phosphate calcium is not easily digested and is a powerful alkalizing substance (TUMS™ is made of calcium carbonate). This is the opposite of what is required to fix a broken stomach. Milk does have high protein, which raises acid levels. However, this momentary benefit is insufficient compared to its overall alkalizing effects. (See Part 3: *The Heartburn and the HCl paradox*).

WHAT ABOUT REAL BUTTER? Butter is acceptable when used sparingly. Feel free to have a small pat on your vegetables.

CAN MILK SUBSTITUTES FROM PLANTS BE USED? Yes, but only if they contain less than 10% of the RDA of calcium. Unfortunately, the dairy-free product industry knows all too well that people expect to get a high amount of calcium from their milk. So, when consumers are deciding to switch to a dairy-free option, food companies make their choice much easier by adding 45% of the RDA of calcium per cup (usually the acid-dampening carbonate form). This amount equals ¾ of a TUMS tablet and 50% more total calcium than is found in cow's milk. Be sure to read the labels.

AVOID ABRASIVE FOODS

Do not eat the following:

- Salads (all lettuces, kale, and spinach in their raw form)
- Seeds
- Popcorn
- Corn chips
- Granola
- Dried fruit
- Cereal
- Handfuls of nuts (nut butters are acceptable)

Patients often complain that they will not get enough nutrients if they don't eat salads. This can be true in the short term. However, their nutrient absorption ability has likely been long compromised because of intestinal inflammation, which the *Gentle GI Diet* will correct. **A MUCH WIDER VARIETY OF FOODS WILL ONCE AGAIN BE ACCEPTABLE FOR CONSUMPTION IN 3 TO 6 WEEKS.**

AVOID YEAST-PROMOTING & IRRITATING FOODS

One of the most important steps to overcoming chronic intestinal and systemic candida or other yeast infections is to acidify the stomach and the upper digestive tract. Foods that alkalize must be avoided and include:

- Sugar (very small amounts)
- Soda
- Baking soda — soda breads or sweet breads
- Sweet fruits (small amounts are okay, berries are okay)
- Baker's yeast
- Brewer's yeast
- Alcohol

Foods that irritate the stomach lining itself, alkalize the stomach's digestive juices, or promote intestinal yeast overgrowth must be avoided. Irritating foods differ from person to person but include:

- Spicy foods
- Black pepper, garlic, raw onions
- Tomato sauce
- Coffee and caffeinated drinks (Not to worry. Just use your CoffeeShack Gold Member points for something decaf).

SIX WAYS CHOCOLATE HURTS

Chocolate is one of the most hormonally disruptive chemicals around. "But I heard that dark chocolate is good for you." I have heard it too. Just Google *health benefits of chocolate* and you will find plenty of articles extolling the advantages of this "super-food." Careful, things are not always as they seem.

SURPRISE! ADVERTISERS DON'T GIVE THE WHOLE TRUTH

When marketers want to sell you a product, they will promote the positives and downplay the negatives. There are hundreds of chemicals in chocolate. All a marketer must do is highlight the benefits of the "good" chemicals. Notice I did not say the benefits of the chocolate. I said the benefits of the chemicals in the chocolate. The individual chemicals do not matter. The entire food is what must be evaluated. Let me give you an example.

DRINK SODA TO STAY HYDRATED

Water is essential to life. Healthy people drink half their body weight or more in ounces of water per day. Soda contains 90% water. And diet soda contains 99% water. So, why bother with those fancy bottles filled with filtered or spring water? To achieve your recommended daily intake of water, simply consume six to eight cans of regular or diet soda!

Does that sound like good health advice to you? It is exactly what marketers do with chocolate, milk, wine, and every other food they want you to consume. Here are six examples of complaints from patients that are often directly related to the ingestion of chocolate:

1. **CHRONIC NON-TRAUMATIC HIP PAIN IN WOMEN** – Chocolate has a profound influence on the hormonal system. One common effect is sluggish metabolism of the estrogen hormones. The muscles of the hormonal system, such as the piriformis, are strong stabilizers of the hip joint. Therefore, with too much negative influence from the presence of chocolate, the hip muscles become turned off (inhibited), which ironically feels like a tightness, and the joint itself becomes unstable. A constant dull ache with occasional sharp stabbing pain often follows. Many times, these pains can feel worse when getting up from a seated position or when in bed, so much so that they can keep you awake.

2. **SUDDEN ONSET SEVERE NECK PAIN (CHOCOLATE NECK SYNDROME)** – I have seen this dozens of times. Usually the scenario goes like this: "I don't know what happened. I didn't do anything crazy. I just woke up like this." Then I ask if they had some chocolate last evening? Around 70% of the time the answer is, "yes." In many cases these patients are also going through a season of remarkably high stress, which exacerbates the chemical reactions from chocolate, making things more painful.

   - The mechanism for the neck pain has to do with a calcium / magnesium imbalance. Usually calcium is low (or poorly processed), and magnesium suddenly swings high. Chocolate is full of magnesium (65% of the RDA in a 100g bar). If eaten in a high enough quantity when this imbalance is present, the parathyroid glands will kick into high gear to regulate the calcium deficiency by secreting parathyroid hormone (pulls out usable calcium from the bones). This emergency measure causes the muscles related to the parathyroid gland to "freak out" either by becoming inhibited or facilitated, resulting in a strong pain response with a decreased range of motion. Which muscles? The muscles related to the parathyroid gland are the levator scapulae, located, you guessed it, on the back of neck.

3. **MIGRAINE HEADACHES** – Chocolate is a strong booster of serotonin and a disruptor of estrogen metabolism. Migraine headaches are many times an emergency measure by the body to reduce elevated serotonin levels in the brain. Changes in estrogen levels make the serotonin receptors in the brain more sensitive, magnifying the painful effects of elevated serotonin. As many will attest, migraines are more common near the initiation of the menstrual cycle when estrogen levels are fluctuating. To alleviate migraines, it is often necessary to reduce serotonin and detox estrogen at the same time. Eating chocolate prevents this from happening.

4. **POOR ESTROGEN METABOLISM** – Chocolate has a profound disruptive effect on the female hormonal cycle because of its influence on estrogen metabolism. Heavy bleeding, breast tenderness, irritability, and painful cramping are common. Dairy products do the same thing because of the same calcium/magnesium mechanism, but coming from the calcium side, rather than the magnesium side (this teeter-totter is discussed in STEP 5).

5. **SLEEP DISRUPTIONS** – All of the hormonal and mineral imbalances created by chocolate can initiate, or contribute to, an adrenaline-based blood sugar-swinging physiology with all its many symptoms. Insomnia in its various forms is one of the most common.

6. **CHRONIC MUSCLE AND/OR JOINT PAIN** – Anything that forces the liver to work hard can lead to muscle or joint pain. An adrenaline-based physiology creates metabolic and inflammatory by-products that slow down detoxification in the liver. Pain can manifest in the soft tissues as the chemical agents build up in muscles and organs.

   Pain can also originate in the joints because sulfur is hoarded by the liver as a necessary agent of sulfation detoxification. This means that the joints do not receive adequate amounts of sulfur for soft tissue repair (soft tissues like ligaments and tendons are made from glucose and sulfur).

If you are experiencing any of these issues just mentioned, avoiding chocolate and dairy products will likely help (yes, even the "small" square or two of chocolate eaten every night can create these problems).

GENTLE AI DIET (6 WEEKS TO A LIFETIME)

The *Gentle AI Diet* is a much stricter diet required for those who suffer from an autoimmune disease or debilitating chronic illness. It is also for those who have been on the *Gentle GI Diet* for 21 days and still have noticeable digestive issues.

The *Gentle AI Diet* should be followed for at least six weeks. With certain autoimmune diseases, some form of the *Gentle AI Diet* may be necessary for the rest of your life.

The *Master Food List* below can still be used as a shopping list. However, be sure to avoid any foods marked with double asterisks (**).

There are many great cookbooks available to make this process much less painful. Here are two of my favorites:

The Autoimmune Protocol Made Simple Cookbook by: Sophie Van Tiggelen

Fed and Fit by: Cassy Joy Garcia

DO NOT EAT FOODS CONTAINING GLUTEN

Gluten is a protein found in many grains including wheat, barley, and rye. It is common in foods, such as bread, pasta, pizza, and cereal. People with celiac disease who eat gluten experience a painful and destructive immune reaction that damages their intestinal tracts and other tissues of their body. Current estimates suggest that up to 1% of the population has true Celiac disease.[16] For them, a gluten-free diet is a medical necessity. However, up to 40% of people have gluten intolerance. They too should avoid gluten products until the GI tract is fully healed.

BUT I DON'T HAVE CELIAC DISEASE SO I CAN EAT GLUTEN, RIGHT?

Maybe not. The anecdotal evidence demonstrating gluten as a cause of highly reactive inflammatory responses from the immune system, even in non-celiac people, is piling up.

What you need to know is whether your immune system is making antibodies not just to the gluten protein, but to any of its portions, or any other similar proteins through what is known as cross-reactivity. If it is, pain, inflammation, and tissue destruction will follow.

Most doctors only check for alpha gliadin antibodies—the portion of gluten most associated with celiac disease. Many times, this test comes back negative. The patient, believing they are in the clear, continues to eat gluten while their health deteriorates.

THERE ARE THIRTY-TWO DIFFERENT GLUTEN FRACTIONS AND TWENTY-EIGHT CROSS-REACTIVE FOODS that can be tested for antibodies. Beyond this, **gluten has protein sequences that are identical to the protein sequences in the brain, the thyroid, the pancreas, and other tissues in the body.**[17] If antibodies have been made to any of these, eating gluten could cause an immune system attack on otherwise healthy organs and tissues.

To find out if you are cross-reacting with gluten, you can ask your doctor to perform a blood test from Cyrex Laboratories called, *Gluten-Associated Cross-Reactive Foods and Foods Sensitivity Panel*.

NIGHTSHADES CAUSE PAIN

Those with gluten antibodies often feel the immune system's wrath after eating only a tiny amount of this protein. This is because nearly all pain-causing inflammatory chemicals are the consequence of the immune system attacking and destroying what it has deemed a hostile invader, or antigen. This fact is true for far more foods than just gluten.

Nightshades vegetables (tomatoes, potatoes, peppers, etc.) are another recognized food group to do so. But I am here to tell you that I have seen dozens of "healthy" foods cause these same pain patterns. This is why it is always wise to rotate foods in the diet, especially the ones you eat most often and the ones you have eaten for years.

FOODS TO AVOID TO CALM INFLAMMATION

- All grains such as oats, rice, corn, and wheat
- All milk-based products from all animal types except for butter
- Eggs from all animal types
- Legumes such as beans and peanuts
- Nuts
- Nightshade vegetables (tomatoes, eggplants, peppers, and potatoes)
- All sugars including sugar replacements (except for the occasional use of honey)
- All oils (except for avocado, coconut, ghee, and olive)
- Food additives
- Alcohol

WHY NO GRAINS?

There are several naturally gluten-free grains including: amaranth, buckwheat, corn, millet, rice, and quinoa. However, until you know for sure which grains you can eat, avoid them all. Why? Grains are highly cross-reactive with gluten, meaning they have also been tagged with antibodies and will cause the same inflammatory effect as gluten when eaten.

ADDING FOODS BACK IN (AFTER 6 WEEKS)

After following these guidelines for six weeks, some of you may be able to add more foods back into your diet. Begin with rice, eggs, potatoes, and nut butters. I strongly recommend repeating the *Gluten-Associated Cross-Reactive Foods and Foods Sensitivity Panel* before adding in any other foods.

FODMAP DIET

If after six weeks fruits, sugars, or honey still bother your digestive system, and/or you know you have IBS, then follow the rules of the FODMAP diet.

FODMAP stands for fermentable oligosaccharides, disaccharides, monosaccharides, and polyols. In simpler terms, FODMAPs are certain forms of short-chain carbohydrates (sugars) found in foods. When eaten in excess, they may not be digested or absorbed well and could become overly fermented by bacteria in your intestinal tract. This produces hydrogen gas and causes digestive symptoms in sensitive individuals. FODMAPs also draw liquid into your intestine, which may cause diarrhea. Although not everyone is sensitive to FODMAPs, this is very common among people with irritable bowel syndrome (IBS).

The FODMAPs include:

- FRUCTOSE: fruits, honey, and high fructose corn syrup

- LACTOSE: (some dairy products have low levels of lactose and are acceptable)

- FRUCTANS (inulin): wheat, onion, and garlic

- GALACTANS: beans, lentils, and legumes like soy

- POLYOLS: sweeteners containing sorbitol, mannitol, xylitol, maltitol, and stone fruits, such as avocado, apricots, cherries, nectarines, peaches, and plums

For more information on the FODMAP diet see:

https://www.ibsdiets.org/fodmap-diet/fodmap-food-list/

SOURCES OF GLUTEN

Going gluten free and grain free will undoubtedly be difficult at first, especially if you regularly eat fast food and processed food. This is further complicated by the many hidden sources of gluten, like the ones listed below. Thankfully, the list of gluten-free food options available in the grocery store continues to grow.

BAKING POWDER: Some brands of baking powder contain gluten. Look for a brand that says "gluten-free" or make your own. Here is the recipe: l/4 cup baking soda + 1/2 cup cream of tartar + 1/2 cup arrowroot powder. Place ingredients into a glass jar with a lid and shake gently. Store jar in a cool, dry place.

BEER: Beer and ale are fermented and contain gluten from the wheat and barley from which they are made.

BREAD: Bread made with flours such as whole wheat flour, white flour, unbleached flour, all-purpose flour, spelt flour, kamut flour, barley flour, and rye flour all contain gluten as well as many sprouted breads.

BROWN RICE SYRUP: Some brands use barley although Lundberg Brown Rice syrup is gluten-free.

CANDY: Wheat flour or starch may be used to prevent sticking during the shaping and handling of candy.

CARAMEL COLOR: May contain gluten in the form of wheat starch or malt syrup if it was foreign made.

CEREAL: Breakfast cereals are often made from wheat, spelt, kamut, barley, and rye or contain malt flavoring,

CITRIC ACID: Citric acid can be fermented from wheat, corn, molasses, or beets. It may contain gluten if it is imported from other countries that may use wheat.

COFFEE: Some brands of instant coffee and some flavored coffee drinks use wheat as a flavor carrier.

DAIRY PRODUCTS: Some dairy products contain modified food starch which may contain gluten.

DEXTRIN: In the U.S. dextrin is usually made from com or tapioca, but it can be made from wheat.

FLAVORINGS: Natural flavorings are usually gluten-free, though some flavorings for meat may contain wheat.

FLOUR: Make sure all flours say gluten-free.

GRAINS: The cereal grains wheat, spelt, kamut, barley, bulgur wheat, and rye all contain gluten.

MALT: Malt may be made from barley and therefore could contain gluten.

MALTODEXTRIN: In the U.S., maltodextrin cannot contain gluten unless it is declared on the ingredient label.

MEAT: Fillers are used in many processed meats including sausages, luncheon meats, and hot dogs and need to be avoided on a gluten-free diet. Also be sure to avoid self-basting turkeys.

MISO: Look for a miso that uses rice koji and is labeled "gluten-free."

MODIFIED FOOD STARCH: Can contain gluten if imported.

NON-DAIRY MILK: Look for a brand that is labeled "gluten-free."

OATMEAL: Oats are naturally gluten-free although most oats sold in the U.S. may be contaminated with gluten during harvesting, processing, or packaging. Look for certified gluten-free oats.

PACKAGED DESSERT MIXES: Pudding mixes, cake mixes, frosting mixes, and cake decorations all usually contain gluten. Look for the word gluten-free on the label.

SEASONINGS: Packaged seasoning mixes made from a combination of spices and herbs usually contain wheat flour as a carrier that may not be declared on the label.

SOUPS AND SOUP MIXES: Many packaged or canned soups use wheat as a thickener. Bouillon cubes often use wheat as a binder.

SOY SAUCE: Soy sauce contains wheat. Look for wheat-free tamari as a replacement instead.

VEGETABLE STARCH: Vegetable starch or vegetable protein on the ingredient label could mean it came from peanuts, rice, com, soy, or wheat.

VINEGAR: Distilled vinegar made from grains is safe to eat because gluten cannot survive the distillation process though malt vinegar contains gluten and is not safe to eat. Wine vinegars, brown rice vinegars, and apple cider vinegar are all gluten-free and are safe to consume.

YEAST: Nutritional yeast or brewer's yeast is a by-product of the brewing industry that may contain gluten. Baking yeast used to make bread rise is gluten-free. However, up to three-quarters of gluten-sensitive people are often yeast sensitive as well.

MASTER FOOD LIST

If you are following the *Gentle AI Diet,* foods marked with double asterisks (**) are to be avoided.

SEASONINGS

Daily

Spicy foods can make existing inflammatory reactions in the body much worse, especially hot peppers, chai teas, and curry. Keep it simple. **These herbs are from the nightshade family.

- ☐ Basil
- ☐ Black and white Pepper
- ☐ **Cayenne Pepper
- ☐ **Chili Powder
- ☐ Cumin
- ☐ Curry Powder
- ☐ Garam Masala
- ☐ Herbs
- ☐ Italian Seasoning
- ☐ Oregano
- ☐ **Red Pepper Flakes
- ☐ Sea salt
- ☐ Thyme

- ☐ Allspice
- ☐ Cardamom
- ☐ Cilantro
- ☐ Cinnamon
- ☐ Cloves
- ☐ Dill
- ☐ Ginger
- ☐ Nutmeg
- ☐ **Paprika
- ☐ Parsley
- ☐ Rosemary
- ☐ Sage
- ☐ Turmeric

FATS

Daily

Fats play a HUGE role in a healthy diet. Fats make up a huge chunk of your calorie intake so make sure you are taking in plenty of healthy fats!

- ☐ Avocado Oil
- ☐ Butter (grass fed)
- ☐ Cocoa Butter
- ☐ Coconut Oil
- ☐ Duck Fat
- ☐ Ghee
- ☐ Lard
- ☐ Macadamia Oil

- ☐ MCT Oil
- ☐ Olive Oil
- ☐ Palm Shortening
- ☐ Red Palm Oil
- ☐ Sesame Oil
- ☐ Tallow
- ☐ Walnut Oil

MEATS / EGGS / FISH

Daily

All meats, fish and shellfish are acceptable if they are well-cooked to a soft consistency or are medium rare in the case of red meats—think rotisserie chicken, salmon, **eggs (of any animal), prime rib, etc. Also, find the highest quality meats possible. Local, grass fed, and wild caught are best. **Processed meats can contain several additives, preservatives and flavor enhancers that are detrimental to your health. These should be avoided.**

- ☐ Beef
- ☐ Bison
- ☐ Chicken
- ☐ Clams
- ☐ Cod
- ☐ Crab
- ☐ Deer
- ☐ Duck
- ☐ Elk
- ☐ Goat
- ☐ Goose
- ☐ Lamb
- ☐ Mahi mahi

- ☐ Moose
- ☐ Oyster
- ☐ Pheasant
- ☐ Pork
- ☐ Quail
- ☐ Red snapper
- ☐ Salmon
- ☐ Sheep
- ☐ Shrimp
- ☐ Turkey
- ☐ Veal
- ☐ Wild boar
- ☐ Wild turkey

VEGETABLES

Daily

All kinds so long as they are well cooked.

Make it your goal to have ½ of your plate filled with cooked green and colored vegetables!

- ☐ Arugula
- ☐ Artichokes
- ☐ Asparagus
- ☐ **Bell Peppers
- ☐ Bok Choy
- ☐ Broccoli
- ☐ Brussels Sprouts
- ☐ Butterhead Lettuce
- ☐ Cabbage
- ☐ Cauliflower
- ☐ Celery
- ☐ Chard
- ☐ Chicory Greens

- ☐ Chives
- ☐ Cucumber
- ☐ Dandelion greens
- ☐ **Eggplant
- ☐ Endives
- ☐ Fennel
- ☐ Garlic
- ☐ Kale
- ☐ Kohlrabi
- ☐ **Onion
- ☐ Squash
- ☐ Zucchini

41

ROOT VEGETABLES

Three to five times a week

These starchy foods are satisfying for the palate and can be eaten regularly in small amounts (no more than ¼ of your plate). Rotate these with your grains.

☐ Beets
☐ Carrots
☐ **Potato (white)

☐ Potato (sweet)
☐ Radishes
☐ Turnips
☐ Yams

FRUITS

Three times a week

Eat cooked fruit and skinless (larger fruits), berries and avocados. Always eat them with protein. Many fruits are higher glycemic and affect your blood sugar which must be stabilized. Some small amounts of berries are okay but watch how much you eat. Fruits generally have higher sugar content which is what we're trying to avoid.

☐ Avocado
☐ Blackberry
☐ Blueberry
☐ Cherry
☐ Cranberry

☐ Lemon
☐ Lime
☐ Olive
☐ Raspberry
☐ Strawberry

GRAINS

Three times a week
(Rotated with root vegetables)

If you are trying to lose weight, keep your total carbohydrates under 50grams (about two slices of sandwich bread per day). All grains count as your ¼ plate of carbohydrates. It is easy to eat too much bread or pasta—be extra careful. Remember, gluten products can be highly inflammatory for some people. If you are not sure that you are safe to eat gluten, stick to gluten free (GF).

☐ Rice (mostly white)
☐ Quinoa
☐ **Oats
☐ **Wheat
☐ Gluten-free products

GLUTEN-FREE FLOURS

Three times a week

All GF flours are acceptable. Be cautious. Many are made with nuts, which do cause problems for some if eaten daily. Listen to your body to make sure it is not reacting negatively (bloating, gas, pain, pressure). If it is, assume that your most recently consumed food(s) is harmful to you and avoid it.

LEGUMES / BEANS

Three times a week

Some people are sensitive to the lectins in beans, which causes them to bloat or experience other bowel discomfort. **If you have joint pain, then avoid this category except for green beans and peas.** Soaking for a few hours, draining the water, and then cooking is helpful.

- ☐ Green beans
- ☐ Navy beans
- ☐ Fava beans
- ☐ Pinto beans
- ☐ Kidney beans
- ☐ Chickpeas
- ☐ Lentils (soaking not required)
- ☐ Peanuts (as nut butter)

NUTS

Three to five times a week

Nut butters are acceptable, but raw nuts and nuts with skins are to be avoided for three weeks. Rotate all nut butters and take a day off from all nuts every three days.

- ☐ Almond butter
- ☐ Cashew butter
- ☐ Sunflower butter
- ☐ Peanut butter

SHAKES

Twice a week

Non-chocolate egg or plant-based (not whey)

These are a good twice-a-week option so long as there is plenty of protein mixed in. A straight fruit smoothie is far too disruptive to the blood sugar system. Remember this big rule: have protein in all meals. Also, only add a small amount of kale, spinach, or other vegetables to your shake. Eat these cooked primarily.

SOUPS

Three to five times a week

These must be dairy free. Tomato-based soups can also be inflammatory for many people. Stick to bone or vegetable broth soups instead. You can also drink bone broth between meals as a part of a snack. Keep the seasonings simple: salt, pepper, and herbs. Be sure to add plenty of meat and vegetables.

MISCELLANEOUS

Additional foods that are permitted to eat

- ☐ Carob
- ☐ Coconut Butter
- ☐ Cod Liver Oil (Fish Oil)
- ☐ Fish Sauce (check ingredients)
- ☐ Gelatin (as a powder or from bone broth)
- ☐ Gluten Free Tamari Sauce or Coconut Aminos
- ☐ Hot Sauce (check ingredients)
- ☐ Mayonnaise (made with good oils - see list of oils)
- ☐ Monk Fruit or Luo Han Guo Sweetener
- ☐ Mustard
- ☐ Pickles
- ☐ Shredded Coconut
- ☐ Stevia (small amounts if necessary)
- ☐ Vanilla Extract
- ☐ Vinegars (apple cider, balsamic, red wine, and white wine vinegars)

STEP 4: REIGNITE

BURN FAT ONCE AGAIN BY WAKING UP YOUR SLEEPING METABOLISM

If you have had trouble losing weight after starving yourself and exercising regularly, you know that something is wrong with the calories in/calories out equation.[18] Once again, adrenaline dominance is at fault.

More specifically, after years of living with the imbalances caused by fight-or-flight, your metabolism has been trained to rely on fast-acting, low-energy sugars for fuel rather than high-energy fat. Long-term, this stubborn state does more than make you less shapely. It promotes functional illnesses of all kinds.

Thankfully, alongside the *50 FIX Plan*, a technique called *Glucose-Guided Eating (GGE)*, is the missing piece of the puzzle for many. With GGE and the rest of the *50 FIX Plan* you now have the means to reignite a dampened metabolism.

But before we dive into the details, let's briefly discuss the basic principles of losing fat.

BURN UP YOUR BLOOD GLUCOSE FIRST

To burn stored body fat, you must first deplete other forms of energy in your bloodstream and in the liver. These are fuels such as alcohols, ketones, glucose, and essential fatty acids. Blood sugar is the energy that will be burned up first, and even more so during times of fight-or-flight.

As you deplete blood glucose, it is refilled from the glycogen stores in your liver and muscles (glycogen is the fancy name for the body's stored form of glucose). Then, once glycogen is getting low, the body starts working on the fat in your blood for energy. **Finally, when the glucose and fat in your blood are diminished, your body will begin burning its stored fat.**

What all this means is, if you eat your next meal before your blood glucose levels have gone below a certain point (your baseline) then your energy reserves are not being tapped into and you have an energy excess. In this scenario, your body has no choice but to store the excess as fat. Long-term energy excesses pack on the pounds and do great internal damage as well. This is now an ENERGY TOXICITY.

And here is a terrible reality for some...Depending on your metabolic efficiency, you can store fat from an energy excess **even if you are on a low-calorie diet!** This is why measuring your glucose is so important.

PERSONAL FAT THRESHOLD

The amount of fat your body can comfortably store on the outside (your adipose tissue) is known as your *Personal Fat Threshold*. Once your body exceeds this threshold the fuels in your bloodstream like glucose levels, ketones, and free fatty acids, start to build up or worse.

If stored energy levels continue to rise, visceral fat is deposited in and around your vital organs like your liver, pancreas, and heart. Now metabolic momentum is pressing you well beyond functional illness toward obesity, metabolic syndrome (diabetes + heart disease), cancer, and a host of other unwanted horribles.

So, yes, the 'muffin tops' or 'jelly bellies' we notice on the outside motivate us to lose weight. And this is good. But the visceral fat we don't see on the inside turns out to be the true disfigurement.

WEIGHT LOSS RULES

RULE #1 DO ALL THE STEPS OF THE 50 FIX PLAN!

Each of the 10 STEPS of the *50 FIX Plan* work together to calm adrenaline dominance throughout the body. This means if you do the *Gentle GI Diet* but do not take your supplements, or drink your water, or get quality sleep, you could sabotage your efforts. Likewise, you need to use and make muscles to burn fat. STEP 6: *Restercise* helps you do it the right way. The whole *50 FIX* team needs to be on the field for you to score your health goals!

RULE #2 DO NOT OVEREAT

As I observe those who live long and healthy lives, no matter how they eat they usually have one thing in common: they do not overeat. Consequently, these folks are often not overweight and have not irritated their digestive tracts. They are even able to occasionally eat desserts and other less than optimal foods without issue because they enjoy them in small amounts. Eat to feel satisfied, not to feel full.

RULE #3 ONLY 50-75 GRAMS OF CARBS

Minimizing daily carbohydrates is the most common approach to weight loss because it works. Carb overdose is the biggest reason you have a weight loss issue in the first place. There is no RDA for carbs. You can live without them and some of you may need to. Keep it simple: have no more than 50-75 grams of carbohydrates per day.

RULE #4 EAT ONLY FROM THE MASTER FOOD LIST

The *Master Food List* only contains clean, unprocessed foods. Eating these means you are minimizing carbs, sugar, hidden sugars, bad fats, toxins, etc. This is the primary goal—no more spiking and crashing and far less inflammation. Eliminating these will powerfully move you toward a more optimal state of health and vitality.

RULE #5 SNACKS, YES, OR NO?

The answer depends on whether you have hypoglycemia or insulin sensitivity/resistance. In other words, how stable is your blood glucose?

HYPOGLYCEMIA (LOW BLOOD SUGAR) - If you get shaky, lightheaded, or hangry with delayed meals, or you have anxiety, then assume hypoglycemia is present. You should not go more than 2 ½ hours without some food. So, be sure to have good FAT AND PROTEIN SNACKS like those from your sample list in STEP 3. In your case, even if you want to lose weight, DO NOT skip meals for at least 6 WEEKS. Also, start tracking your glucose so you can gauge improvements and know when it is best to eat (see RULE #6).

INSULIN SENSITIVITY/RESISTANCE (HIGH BLOOD SUGAR) – Resistance occurs when a hormone rings a cell's doorbell (receptor site), but no one answers. There is a malfunction. Like when the checkout machine doesn't recognize your debit card even though there is plenty of money in the bank.

Receptor site resistance can happen with any type of hormone—thyroid, sex hormones, insulin, etc.—and usually with more than one at the same time. When it does occur, weight gain is likely.

Insulin resistance can make you feel tired and sluggish especially after eating too many carbohydrates. Therefore, if you do not have any signs of hypoglycemia when you miss meals and you also feel like taking a nap after eating carbs, then YOU SHOULD SKIP SNACKS and move on to RULE #6.

HORMONE RESISTANCE – Hormone resistance is common with weight issues. This is why women start gaining weight at perimenopause. Hormone resistance often makes you feel swollen and painful (particularly the hip joints). If you do not have any issues before or after eating, but you gain weight easily or can't get weight off, then assume you have hormone resistance. Again, NO SNACKS and begin RULE #6.

RULE # 6 GLUCOSE-GUIDED EATING

Glucose-guided eating (GGE) is based off the work of engineer, Marty Kendall. Marty developed *Data Driven Fasting* to help his wife, Monica, who as a young girl, was diagnosed with Type 1 Diabetes (the autoimmune kind).

The great discovery of this method is that to reignite your metabolism, you must first "resensitize" your insulin by having a **proper glucose level before you eat.** Now you will be able to overcome stubborn fat and lose weight. So, if *your* glucose level is too high, then fast a bit longer until it drops into *your* trigger range.

For many years now Marty and his team have guided thousands of people toward their fat loss and blood glucose goals without tracking calories or using a rigid, one size-fits-all fasting window.

I strongly recommend that you take a look at his program or join his masterclass for 30 days to become an expert yourself and join up with a worldwide community.

Visit:

www.datadrivenfasting.com

Here in the *50 FIX Guidebook*, we are going to be piggybacking on Marty's concepts with several important modifications to make sure we address the additional scenarios caused by adrenaline dominance and insulin insensitivity.

THE BENEFITS OF INTERMITTENT FASTING (THE RIGHT WAY)

Fasting gives the entire digestive system a break. Since the processing and absorption of food uses large amounts of energy and resources, just skipping meals from time to time has been shown to result in numerous and profound health benefits.

Fasting promotes longevity, cleans up dysfunctional cells (autophagy), reduces free radicals thereby reducing inflammation and cancer cell proliferation, boosts immunity, regulates proper hunger signals, and spikes growth hormone, which is very important for tissue healing and overall wellbeing.

With all these health bonuses it becomes obvious that fasting should be part of any wellness routine. But there are wrong ways to do things and there are right ways to do things.

Because adrenaline dominance is lurking in the background, how and when you fast from meals is critical for reasons I will now explain.

GLUCOSE-GUIDED EATING

The *Master Food List* from STEP 3 informs you of what to eat; glucose-guided eating (GGE) instructs you when to eat. GGE works by tracking your glucose levels at various times but primarily BEFORE YOU EAT. This is to make sure your glucose levels are not too high. When they are, EATING SHOULD BE POSTPONED.

With GGE you will learn to stretch your mealtimes just a little, but not so much that your body rebels with a FOF response, which is how many become trapped in an endless restrict-binge-restrict cycle.

To get started, all you need is a GLUCOMETER from any drugstore or online and the directions below.

Yes, a continuous glucose monitor would make things much easier, but they can be quite expensive and may bog you down with too much data. Instead, here are the five important numbers we need to know:

THE NUMBERS TO REMEMBER

	NUMBER	ACTION
BASELINE	Your 3-day average morning glucose (Recalculated every week)	Only eat when your glucose is at baseline or below
FEED	If your glucose drops **10+ POINTS BELOW BASELINE**	MUST EAT NOW
FAST	When glucose is **ABOVE BASELINE** (If you must eat, stick to lean protein and greens)	EAT LATER
WHOOPS	If glucose goes **40+ points above baseline** after a meal, you have eaten a No-No food or combo.	Avoid or eat less of the carbohydrate/fat you had at your last meal
TWEAK	When glucose has been **above baseline for >2 hours**	Either the wrong type, or wrong food was eaten. See IMPORTANT below.

	Fasting (mg/dL)	30 minutes after meals (mg/dL)	90-120 minutes after meals (mg/dL)	HbA1C (blood value)
IDEAL	85	<120	<90	4-5.0%
NORMAL	<100	<140	<100	<6%
PRE-DIABETIC	100-146	140-200	Above baseline	6.0% to 6.4%
TYPE 2 DIABETIC	>126	>200	Above baseline	>6.4%

YOUR GOAL

The goal is a baseline around 80-90 mg/dL. Yours may be higher or lower than ideal. If it is, then you have at least one reason weight loss has been difficult.

People with ideal blood sugar balance have a fasting morning glucose around 85 mg/dL. When they eat a quality meal, their levels do not rise more than 30 points and after ninety minutes or so, their levels are back to baseline.

Once your baseline blood glucose is 100 mg/dL or less you can rest assured that while following GGE you will not exceed your *Personal Fat Threshold* and you will be minimizing the risk of diseases associated with energy toxicity and metabolic syndrome.

FINDING YOUR BASELINE

Perform a blood glucose test for three days when you first wake up and before eating. The average of these three numbers is your baseline number. For example:

DAY 1: 105 mg/dL   DAY 2: 99 mg/dL   DAY 3: 107 mg/dL

Average = 103.66 mg/dL

Baseline = 103 mg/dL (always round down)

THE FOUR TIMES TO MEASURE YOUR GLUCOSE

At first you will need to test more often, but don't worry. After you have figured out which carbs or other foods are bothersome and have a day/week meal plan of quality foods that keep your blood sugar in the normal range, you will only need to test as little as once or twice a day.

You can record these four values and your baseline level on each of the 30 tracking sheets in STEP 10.

1. **EVERY MORNING** – To find your BASELINE. Do this within a few minutes of waking.

2. **BEFORE MEALS** - When you feel hungry and begin to think about eating, simply check your blood glucose to validate your hunger and see if you need to FEED or FAST.

3. **THIRTY MINUTES AFTER MEALS** – Do this to check for reactive hypoglycemia and to figure out which foods cause the biggest WHOOPS in your glucose. Usually they are the "white" foods – bread, rice, potato, etc. You will likely do better with one form of carb over another.

4. **TWO HOURS AFTER MEALS** – Testing after two hours helps you to know how quickly your glucose levels are returning to baseline and if your food choices need a TWEAK.

With the four measurements above, you will now know if you are a FEEDER or a FASTER. You will also discover several things: 1) the right time to refuel, 2) if you are craving yummy foods around the house just because they're there, 3) if you are reaching for food to soothe your emotions or relieve boredom, or 4) if you are only eating out of habit (because it's 'lunch time').

IMPORTANT FACTS

- FAST-ACTING CARBS (i.e., white rice, white potato, white bread) will raise your blood glucose quickly. However, they may also come down quickly.

- HIGH-FAT MEALS will help you achieve more stable blood glucose levels, but they may stay elevated and delay when you can eat again.

- Nutritious foods and meals that contain a HIGHER PERCENTAGE OF PROTEIN will give your body what it needs but without excess caloric energy. This allows your body to draw down on its fuel stores. Too much fat and carbs with LOW PROTEIN will keep glucose elevated for too long.

- KEEP A CLOSE EYE ON YOUR GLUCOSE. If it drops below 10-points under baseline it is time to FEED. Otherwise, you may initiate a catabolic response and start to burn up your muscle for fuel.

- Keep a QUALITY SNACK from your *Master Food List* on standby. This will stabilize glucose when needed and keep you from sneaking a low-quality binge food. You CAN drink water, green tea, and other non-caloric beverages during the fast. These often help reduce hunger.

FEEDER OR FASTER OR MIX OF BOTH?

Most people with trouble losing weight will discover their glucose is higher than it should be at the next regular mealtime. They need to wait longer before eating. I call this group the FASTERS. But there is another group who must eat more often because their blood glucose is either too low or is artificially elevated because of fight-or-flight. I call them the FEEDERS.

Neither the FEEDER nor the FASTER may be hungry in the morning and so opt to skip breakfast. But the internal reasons for each group are different.

Both may show a baseline glucose in a good range or even high. For the FASTER, it is likely because of insulin resistance (inefficient transport of glucose into the cell by insulin). For the FEEDER, it is likely because of muscle breakdown, or catabolism.

Chronic fight-or-flight causes the body to break down muscle to make sugar for the nervous system and the brain. This is catabolism, and it is not good.

FEEDERS are the most likely to experience REACTIVE HYPOGLYCEMIA. That is, after they eat, their blood glucose goes up like normal (or high), but soon comes crashing back down to an unhealthy low level (below 70 mg/dL). This sudden drop flips on fight-or-flight and so the muscle-eating cycle continues.

You may be a FEEDER who is experiencing catabolism if you have any of these conditions or symptoms on a semi-regular basis:

- Insomnia (Trouble falling or staying asleep
- Restless leg syndrome
- Anxiety
- POTS
- Hypoglycemia
- Heart palpitations
- Lightheadedness when standing
- Panic attacks
- Shortness of breath
- Sweaty hands and feet

To break this pattern, FEEDERS must intentionally feed their bodies a quality meal (or part of a meal) **within 40 minutes of waking,** and they must also eat **regular healthy snacks.**

There are also times when your body can change from a FEEDER to a FASTER or vice versa, like when life is super stressful, during a time of illness, or with intense exercise.

By the way, EMOTIONAL STRESS can be disruptive to your blood sugar levels FOR DAYS!

Regular checking of your glucose levels in the beginning of GGE will help you know which type of person you are and how to set your schedule.

WHEN TO EAT? - TIMING IS EVERYTHING

Even if you are not eating carbohydrates, your fuel stores (blood glucose and glycogen) are never fully drained. Why is that? Because your body can make glucose from the protein, and even from some of the fat you have eaten. Also, if you are eating very few carbs or protein, your body will quickly turn to your muscles to make glucose especially if you have been in adrenaline dominance. So, when do you eat?

If you are a FEEDER, your body has been trained to pull glucose from your muscles. This means you need to eat as close to when your glucose goes below baseline as possible. The longer you are below your baseline the greater the chance you will turn on FOF and burn up your muscle for fuel!

> NO MATTER WHO YOU ARE,
> ALWAYS EAT IF YOUR GLUCOSE IS
> 10+ POINTS BELOW BASELINE.

WHEN NOT TO EAT?

If your blood glucose is above your baseline number, just wait a little longer until it drops below this point. BUT IF YOU'RE STARVING AND CAN'T WAIT ANY LONGER, you can have a few bites of protein/veggie with very little fat/carb (carbs raise it up, fats keep it up). Within 30 minutes your blood sugar should drop to below baseline. Now it is safe to have your meal.

If you are a FASTER and your glucose is not more than 10 points below your baseline and you are not too hungry, then do not eat. This is how you will lose weight. During this time of fasting, you will begin to use up stored energy and switch over to fat burning.

When it is time to fast, be sure to do so in a calm, restful mode. Don't go to the gym. Don't get on the phone with an energy-stealing person. Don't watch scary movies or intense political shows. Keep your CORE calm for maximum results.

HOW DO I KNOW IF I HAVE EATEN A BAD MEAL?

There are always sneaky carbs. I have patients who can eat two cookies with protein and only see their glucose levels rise 20 or 30 points. But, if they eat a piece of wheat bread, even with a protein meal, their glucose can rise 60 points and take more than two hours to return to normal. You will know if a meal had too many carbohydrates for two reasons:

1. If it raised your blood glucose by more than **40 mg/dL** or,

2. Your blood sugars take **more than 2 hours** to return to baseline. If this happens, be sure to eat less of those carbohydrates, or perhaps fats (see below) in the future.

STEP 5: REPLENISH YOUR TEETER-TOTTERS

USE TEETER-TOTTER SUPPLEMENTS IN THEIR PROPER RATIOS (OR *CORE4POWDER*) TO REPLENISH DEFICIENT CELLS AND TISSUES AND ACHIEVE "MIRACLES"

Below are two supplement prescriptions that can be used to calm fight-or-flight and heal the gut at the same time. Option #1 lists the individual supplement bottles. Option #2 uses **Core4Powder** to replace nine of those bottles. Why these particular nutrients help to calm FOF is detailed in the remainder of STEP 5.

OPTION #1 (MAY VARY BASED ON TEST RESULTS OF NUTRIENTS/METALS)

	Breakfast	Lunch	Dinner	Before Bed
Betaine HCL	1 (500 mg)	1 (500mg)	1 (500mg)	
Potassium Citrate	2 (400mg)		2 (400mg)	
EPA/DHA	1 (1000mg)		1 (1000mg)	
Adrenal Cortex	1 (50mg)	1 (50 mg)		
Electrolyte Drink	1			
B12/B6/5-MTHF/B2	1			
Slippery Elm or Marshmallow Root	1		1	
BCAAs (1000mg)	1			1
L-Glutamine (1000mg)	1			1
Calcium/Magnesium Citrate 1:1 ratio				1-2 (300 mg)
Vitamin D-5000 IU				1
Probiotic (Bifidobiotic-based)				1-2

OPTION #2 (USE CORE4POWDER TO REPLACE SEVERAL DAILY CAPSULES)

	Breakfast	Lunch	Dinner	Before Bed
Core4Powder	1 scoop		1 scoop	
Vitamin D-5000 IU				1
EPA/DHA	1 (1000mg)		1 (1000mg)	
Calcium/Magnesium Citrate 1:1 ratio				1-2 (300 mg)

CORE4POWDER

If taking several nutrients during the day seems daunting, there is always Option #2. After 26+ years of discoveries and experimentation, I have assembled the most needed teeter-totter nutrients to calm fight-or-flight and heal the damage it has caused into a customized powder called, *Core4Powder*. If you were to purchase separately all the ingredients in one scoop of *Core4Powder*, it would be like taking a dose from 7 to 10 other high-quality nutraceutical products.

Visit for more information: **www.Core4Powder.com**

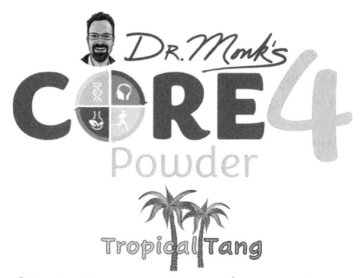

- ✔ Brain Focus
- ✔ Mood & Sleep
- ✔ Glucose Balance
- ✔ Thyroid / Energy
- ✔ Electrolytes
- ✔ Digest & Detox
- ✔ Probiotics
- ✔ Muscle Aminos
- ✔ Hair & Nails
- ✔ Methylated B's

Plus Collagen and MCT Oil!

DIRECTIONS:

Take 1 scoop daily with food, within 40 minutes of waking.
Take an additional scoop as needed to aid with:

Exercise recovery, mild panic symptoms,
stomach discomfort, nausea, trouble sleeping,
or blood sugar swings (hypoglycemia).

Ingredient List
www.Core4Powder.com

Mood and Sleep
Adrenal cortex – 50 mg
Rhodiola – 25 mg
Ashwaganda – 50 mg

Essential Electrolytes
Potassium citrate – 204 mg
Sodium chloride – 75 mg

Bone Macro Minerals
Calcium phosphate/lactate – 42 mg
Magnesium malate – 30 mg

Energy and Focus
B2 Riboflavin-5-phosphate – 20 mg
B3 (inositol Hexaniacinate) – 200 mg
B6 – 5 mg
B12 – 500 mcg
5-MTHF - 0.25 mg

Friendly Probiotics
Bifidobacterium blend
(longus, brevi, lactis, bifidum) – 100 mg
Saccharomyces boulardii – 100 mg

Hair and Nails
Collagen powder – 5400 mg
Biotin 8 mg

Digest and Detox
Betaine HCL – 100 mg
Pancreatin – 50 mg
DGL - 150 mg
Slippery Elm – 100 mg
Beet root – 50 mg
Milk thistle – 25 mg

Muscle Aminos
L-Leucine – 250 mg
L-Valine – 125 mg
L-Isoleucine – 125 mg
L-Glutamine – 500 mg
L-Tyrosine – 200 mg

Glucose Balance
Copper - 0.5 mg
Zinc – 5 mg
Chromium – 50 mcg
Vanadium – 100 mcg
Alpha Lipoic acid – 10 mg

Brain Focus
MCT powder – 500 mg
Potassium iodide – 100 mcg
L - Selenomethionine – 100 mcg

THE TEETER-TOTTER NUTRIENTS

ALL NUTRIENTS MARKED WITH AN "*" ARE PRESENT IN CORE4POWDER.

Many people wonder how it is that they now have nutritional deficiencies when their entire lives they have "been fine." There is no such thing as a perfect food, and many of the staple foods of today are quite imperfect. Eating low nutrition foods devoid of hormetic nutrients strains the digestive process and much more. Since they are not present in the poor-quality food itself, hormetic nutrients must come from the internal reserves. Much like the debt-based society that Americans live in today, the body has borrowed until there is not enough left even to pay the interest. With the regular consumption of processed, low-nutrient, and perhaps GMO foods, the body's bank account of hormetic nutrients is spent to satisfy its daily entitlements. The result is a systemic nutritional deficiency. The nutrients listed below are the most needed to balance the CORE 4 and calm fight-or-flight.

Potassium (K)* / Sodium (Na)* – This teeter-totter is one of the first to become unstable and

its nutrients depleted with adrenaline surges. There are some significant and scary symptoms related directly to K/Na depletion such as heart palpitations and high or low blood pressure. Another reason the K/Na teeter-totter is first on my list is because potassium is used to control acid-base disturbances in the blood. When too acidic, potassium will move from inside the cell out into the bloodstream and do the opposite when too alkaline.

Medical doctors often get nervous when patients are taking potassium. The reason is one of the most common groups of medicines prescribed today are those designed to reduce high blood pressure. Most of these medicines are potassium sparing. That is, they function by preventing potassium from leaving the body. That is a big clue as to the real cause of the high blood pressure in the first place—the patient needed potassium. However, taking potassium above a few hundred milligrams while on blood pressure medicine (BPM), or certain diuretics, may damage the heart or kidneys. That is why the medical doctors fear it. In reality, taking potassium apart from BPM will often reduce high blood pressure while also improving the status of calcium and magnesium in the body, which helps to prevent osteoporosis and kidney stones.[19] So, high blood pressure patients, who have been restricted from potassium by their doctors, are missing the calcium/magnesium benefits as well. In most instances, it would be much better for those with high blood pressure to drop the BPM and take potassium instead (with your doctor's permission of course).

My patients, who are not on BPMs routinely take 600 to 1200mg per day or more of potassium. Surprisingly, it is now recommended that all people consume 4700mg of potassium.[20] The average intake of potassium among adults is less than 3000 mg. According to these numbers everyone you know is potassium deficient. And do not think you will catch up by eating bananas. They only have around 250 mg of potassium each. The good news is, you do not need thousands of milligrams of additional potassium per day, or any mineral for that matter, for reasons I give in the *Betaine HCl* paragraphs below.

Calcium (Ca)* / Magnesium (Mg)* – Calcium imbalances are very common with adrenaline

surges because of low hydrochloric acid levels in the stomach resulting in "bound" calcium in the blood.

The poorly absorbed bound calcium causes anxiety, constipation, muscle spasms, headaches, heart palpitations, trouble falling asleep, bone spurs, increased joint degeneration, and kidney stones. To alleviate these issues, people have turned to magnesium with good success in some cases. The reason for their improvement? The Teeter-Totter Effect. By adding magnesium, the teeter-totter between calcium and magnesium becomes more balanced, but not in an optimal range. Now, they are both temporarily elevated in the body.

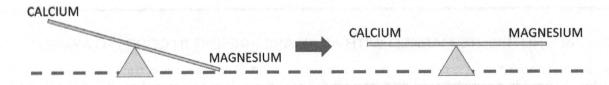

From high calcium, normal magnesium, to both elevated

In this state, some noticeable symptom resolution will occur such as better bowel function, and decreased muscle spasms, but this is a stopgap and does not address the primary imbalance of high bound calcium. Worse yet, poor physiological and metabolic states become established, assuring greater health consequences in the future. Instead, establishing normal levels of free calcium (and magnesium) is the goal. This is done by making sure the stomach has ample quantities of HCl.

Hydrochloric acid (taken as Betaine HCl)* — In *PART 3: The Digestive Tract* I explain
why correcting low stomach acid (hypochlorhydria) is foundational because of the cascade of imbalances low stomach acid creates. Fixing HCl is a necessary first step because **without appropriate levels of HCl, minerals cannot be properly absorbed, and proteins are not fully broken down.** Therefore, a complete health recovery is not possible without the necessary amount of essential minerals and the full complement of amino acids that come from proteins.

HCl is usually packaged as Betaine HCl (taking straight HCl would be a very unpleasant experience and one you would only do once). The betaine portion stabilizes the HCl for use in a capsule. Betaine is also called trimethylglycine, and functions very closely with choline, folic acid, vitamin B12, and a form of the amino acid methionine known as S-adenosylmethionine (SAMe). All of these are "methyl donors." They carry and donate methyl molecules to facilitate many other essential intracellular processes and promote detoxification.

Adrenal Cortex* / DHEA – Adrenaline is the gas pedal for the sympathetic nervous system and
the hormone cortisol is the brake. In prolonged stress, the brakes are worn down to the rotors. Therefore, putting on some new pads is a must. I have historically done this with a glandular product called adrenal cortex. The cortex is the outer part of the adrenal gland and is where cortisol is manufactured. Supplying this product signals the body to begin cortisol restoration, which is a delicate process that cannot be rushed.

Those with fully exhausted adrenal glands are not able to tolerate the gentle push from adrenal cortex. Instead, I use DHEA. This is a short-term hormone needed for only two or three months. By then enough healing has occurred to now allow for the use of adrenal cortex.

It should be noted that there are many exceptional adaptogenic herbs that are very helpful for managing the fight-or-flight response. My favorites are rhodiola and ashwaganda, both of which calm adrenaline and its cousin, noradrenaline, and help with energy and mood. These are included in *Core4Powder*.

Stomach Soothers* / H-Pylori Killers — Some who need HCl, may experience a sensation of burning. This is because the stomach lining is too irritated and sensitive to use the necessary HCl. It could be that the tissue is simply overworked from too much mechanical stress, or an infection could be present.

As explained in *PART 3: Helicobacter Pylori and Ulcers,* a bacterium in the stomach of most people, called H-Pylori, causes ulcers and pain. HCl should not be taken with ulcers. Instead, using herbal products to get rid of the H-Pylori infection is the best course of action. Then, when the lining of the stomach has healed, HCl supplementation should begin.

One of the best ingredients to fix the H-Pylori infection is berberine, a bright yellow compound found in herbs like goldenseal, golden thread, Oregon grape root, and barberry.

Along with berberine, stomach soothing agents can be taken at the same time including marshmallow root, slippery elm, licorice root, and aloe vera.

Enzymes — As powerful as enzymes are, they are usually not the first thing I use for digestive support. In fact, some types of enzymes can irritate the pancreas (the organ that makes most of our digestive enzymes) or the gut itself.

There are two categories of enzymes. The first comes from the pancreas and includes those that digest fat (lipase), carbohydrate (amylase) and protein (protease). **The protein digesting, or proteolytic enzymes, are the ones that should be avoided by those with gluten sensitivity** or significant intestinal lining inflammation. They should also avoid bromelain. Instead, these people should supplement with enzymes made in the gut wall itself called brush border enzymes.

Brush border enzymes include amylase, cellulase, invertase, and lactase. Intestinal damage from an inflamed and leaky gut can reduce and destroy the brush border (microvilli) and its enzyme-making ability. If you experience bloating after eating, anemia, weight loss, and other symptoms of malabsorption, then these enzymes are the better choice for you. Plant-based enzymes are also much safer for those with inflamed intestines.

After being on HCl for weeks or months, then it may be time to add in enzymes for additional food digestion and gut healing; bile salts for gallbladder support may also be helpful at that time. There are HCl combination products that include these additional ingredients. Just be careful to choose the correct form of enzymes.

B12* / B6* / Folic Acid (as 5-MTHF*) — Low HCl, along with its other many deleterious effects, leads to a deficiency in vitamin B12. The reason is, specialized cells in the stomach lining called parietal cells, are responsible for the production of HCl and also make a substance called intrinsic factor – a glycoprotein. Intrinsic factor is necessary for the absorption of vitamin B12 from food. This critical B-vitamin helps with energy and detoxification via methylation. Therefore, people with low HCl also have low B12 and feel very tired (which is why they often need B12 injections). B12 deficiency in turn leads to imbalances in vitamin B6 and folic acid (B9). These falling dominos soon knock iron, copper, and zinc out of balance as well.

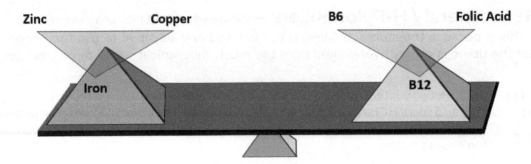

In my experience correcting these two teeter-totters at the same time has been a game changer. Doing so requires individual nutrients, NOT B-COMPLEXES, OR MULTIVITAMINS.

From the cascade of negative events described above, you can now understand why low hydrochloric acid levels are one of the major causes of anemia (the B12 or iron-based kind). Anemia, of course, directly causes systemic health problems because the essential nutrient oxygen is no longer being efficiently utilized in the body by the red blood cells.

Iron, Copper*, Zinc* — These three minerals are critical for hormonal balance, neurotransmitter flow, liver and cellular detoxification, and proper oxygen utilization in the body for energy. Furthermore, depleted iron results in anemia, depleted zinc results in immune dysfunction, and low copper can contribute to poor dopamine metabolism, and thyroid problems.

Estrogen / Progesterone — The balance between these two hormones is so fragile in the presence of adrenaline surges that they must be evaluated with every female patient. In fact, I will prescribe progesterone to my male patients as well in extreme cases of adrenaline dominance. Why? Because progesterone can be converted to cortisol—the brake for adrenaline—and thereby assist in the restoration of adrenal gland exhaustion.

Getting abnormal estrogen levels back in balance is what needs to happen most often. This is done with the two teeter-totters just mentioned—B12/B6/Folic Acid and Iron/Copper/Zinc—and with a few other nutritional helpers listed below.

Vitamin D / Calcium* — This is one of the best examples of the power of a teeter-totter when it shifts out of balance. I will now describe four different scenarios where **taking vitamin D becomes harmful.** Three have to do with calcium and one has to do with the vitamins A and E.

Calcium is necessary for vitamin D metabolism and utilization by the body and vice versa. So, the person who takes vitamin D and 1) has low calcium levels or 2) is full of bound, and therefore unusable calcium (as with too much dairy consumption and/or low HCl levels), will **pull calcium from their own bones**. 3) The person who is simply taking too much vitamin D will also pull calcium from their bones causing a state of hypercalcemia, which can lead to kidney stones and/or heart or kidney dysfunction. Finally, 4) since all essential elements within human physiology have partners or counterparts, if D is too high, then it can cause a relative deficiency of either vitamin A or vitamin E. These two vitamins have profound effects on skin, vascular integrity, eyes, and resting muscle tension.

HOW MUCH VITAMIN D SHOULD I HAVE?—From the perspective of a blood test, the optimal range for Vitamin D is between 45 and 55 ng/ml. Many in the natural health field suggest levels higher than this. I don't. I have repeatedly seen, and had to correct, many patients who were taking vitamin D because of low blood test levels who, unknowingly, were making themselves sick, causing rashes, draining their energy, becoming constipated, and suffering from insomnia because their calcium levels were not balanced at the same time. So, even though there was a legitimate clinical reason to take vitamin D, patients were harming themselves by doing so.

BUT MY BLOOD LEVELS ARE FINE—Health professionals can go wrong by assuming a patient's calcium levels are fine because they appear so on a blood test. While the B-vitamins and the fat-soluble vitamins, like vitamin D, will show imbalances more accurately on blood tests, minerals many times do not. This is because the body's highest priority is to have its blood nutrients maintained within a fine range. To make this happen, the bones, muscles, and cells will offer up any excess nutrients for the benefit of the blood.

By the time nutritional imbalances show up in the blood a disease process has already been present for a long time, but not always. Those with osteoporosis many times will have "normal" blood calcium levels.

"But I take calcium with my D." I hear this one a lot. However, taking bad calcium is just as bad as not having enough calcium. Remember, due to low HCl levels in the stomach, calcium is often "bound." In this state, it is useless or even harmful, which is why your kidneys attempt to excrete it.

Coral calcium, which is mostly calcium carbonate, is chalk. This is one of the worst forms of calcium because it is difficult for many people to metabolize due to its high alkalinity and their low stomach acid levels.

Vitamin D / E / A / K – Vitamin D is a fat-soluble vitamin and is balanced with the other fat-soluble vitamins—E, A and K. Imbalances in this category contribute to several muscle, skin, and eye issues. My body is particularly sensitive to irregularities in this teeter-totter. For me, a middle back muscle spasm that lasted for six months was fixed in three days after taking vitamin E. I have found this same issue countless numbers of times in my patients since that discovery, each having similar "miraculous" responses.

SCREEN POISONING—While writing a previous book I used my laptop as a laptop—reclining in bed while I typed. This prolonged electronic bombardment caused significant pain in my feet and a swollen and contorted 4th toe on my right foot. Vitamin A and DHEA were needed to fix this issue and they did so in less than a week. Interestingly, the 4th toe is on the gallbladder acupuncture meridian. The gallbladder is the organ that processes fats, hormones, and the fat-soluble vitamins like vitamin A. This is yet another piece of evidence demonstrating that everything is connected. Now, because we live in a world of electronics, both vitamin A and DHEA are two supplements I regularly use to help those who spend their lives in front of a computer screen.

It should be noted that fat soluble vitamins build up in body tissues and so are not needed forever. Instead, they should be cycled out unless the stress that produced their need (like working every day in front of a computer) is not eliminated.

Tyrosine* / Tryptophan — These are the two amino acids that are required for the synthesis of dopamine and serotonin, respectively. Both, however, have a variety of other critical health-promoting benefits. L-Tyrosine, for instance, is necessary for the manufacture of thyroid hormones. L-Tryptophan can help mood and sleep while acting as a powerful liver detoxifier when yeast overgrowth is present in the gut.

Omega 3 / Omega 6* EFAs — Essential fatty acids (EFAs) such as fish oils, flax seed oil, evening primrose oil and borage oil, are critical for various functions of the body including: dampening inflammation, improving blood vessel health, supporting healthy skin growth, supporting a healthy brain, and proper nervous system function.

It is well recognized that in civilized society, omega 3 deficiency is the norm. However, the ideal ratio of Omega 3 to omega 6 fatty acids required to restore proper balance is constantly debated. I generally see that patients need at least 2000 mg of omega 3 fish oil per day. Some need triple or more, especially if they complain of painful joints, stiffness, dry skin, dandruff, or hormonal imbalances. In children, a higher ratio of DHA to EPA is required especially when addressing learning, memory, and behavioral issues. These common symptoms are exacerbated by the consumption of fried and processed foods, which deplete the body of its essential oils.

Iodine — Iodine is an essential trace element, which is vital for normal growth and development of the body. Around 60% of iodine is stored in the thyroid gland where it plays a vital role in metabolic functions. Iodine along with L-tyrosine are essential for thyroid hormone formation. Other benefits include the removal of toxins and assisting the body in utilizing minerals like calcium and silicon.

Iodine deficiency is a common finding among natural physicians, especially when their patients live inland—away from the coasts—since iodine is naturally absorbed by breathing ocean air. A deficiency of iodine can have serious effects on the body such as depression, irritability, goiter, abnormal weight gain, decreased fertility, coarse hair, constipation, and fatigue.

Vitamins B1 and B2* — B1 (thiamine) and B2 (riboflavin) are opposites regarding nerve transmission, heart function, and blood vessel tone, as well as many other important bodily functions.[21] Thiamine improves the transmission of nerve impulses and increases blood pressure by constricting blood vessels. This is important in certain patients like those who become dizzy when standing.

Riboflavin is often required to help those with elevated blood pressure and stress-related anxiety, since it relaxes nerve impulses and dilates blood vessels. It can also be helpful for restless leg syndrome, eyelid twitching, or muscle spasms. Both B1 and B2 are needed for energy production but must be properly balanced with each other to be effective.

Vitamins B3* and B5 — B3 (Niacin) and B5 (pantothenic acid), like B1 and B2, have opposing and complementary functions in the body. Niacin is the more calming of the two, being useful for lowering cholesterol, easing arthritis pain, boosting brain function, increasing hormone metabolism, and dilating blood vessels. Pantothenic acid stimulates the adrenal glands and is commonly found in many combination-products designed for adrenal repair. In my experience, I rarely use pantothenic acid until the adrenal glands have been mostly rehabilitated, finding instead that B5 can push the adrenals too hard, too fast.

Pantothenic acid, like all B-vitamins, is necessary for proper digestion and utilization of fats, carbohydrates, and proteins. About 85% of dietary B5 is in the form of CoA or phosphopantetheine, which must be converted to pantothenic acid by digestive enzymes in a healthy intestinal lignin (lumen). Therefore, those with a compromised or inflamed digestive system often are deficient in pantothenic acid as well.

Lactobacillus* and Bifidobacterium*

Over 1000 bacteria belonging to more than 500 different species make up our gut microbiome.[22] Their balance is one of the key indicators of overall health but trying to supplement for each individual probiotic is not possible due to their absence from the market. Thankfully, many of the predominant strains are available. In general, the most common small intestine bacteria are Lactobacilli, whereas the most common large intestine bacteria are Bifidobacterium.

Do not just take probiotics and assume that they are always good for you. Many people will have worsening digestive or immune issues from too much of the wrong kind of probiotic. Even the well-known, L. acidophilus can become too prevalent in the small intestine (especially among those who eat salads daily), needing to be counterbalanced with L. rhamnosus. Here is a list of the most common probiotics used in supplement form:

- Saccharomyces boulardii – (a beneficial yeast)
- L. Sporogenes
- L. Acidophilus
- L. Rhamnosus
- L. Plantarum
- L. Casei
- B. Lactis
- B. Longum
- B. Bifidum
- B. Breve

Alpha-lipoic acid (ALA)*

Alpha lipoic acid is an exceptionally versatile nutrient. Being both water and fat soluble, it is able to function in almost any part of the body. ALA is manufactured in the body, but oftentimes not in the amounts necessary to combat adrenaline dominance.

- Is a potent antioxidant which neutralizes harmful free radicals
- Chelates heavy metals out of body tissue
- Enhances the activity of vitamins C and E
- Produces energy in muscles
- Directs calories into energy production
- Helps maintain healthy glucose metabolism
- Supports the nervous system
- Supports healthy liver function
- Promotes nerve cell health
- Directly recycles and extends the metabolic usage of vitamin C, glutathione, and coenzyme Q10, while it indirectly renews vitamin E

Diindolylmethane (DIM)

DIM is a phytonutrient and antioxidant used to help the liver detoxify and metabolize hormones and their waste products. In my experience, DIM works very well alongside a product called, calcium-d-glucarate, to help women with signs of elevated estrogen such as breast tenderness, heavy menstrual bleeding, and uterine cramping.

The immune system (TH-1 and TH-2) – Knowing which way your immune system naturally teeters is very helpful to prevent sickness during changes of the seasons. I regularly have patients who come into the office just to find out whether they need TH-1 or TH-2 support for themselves and their children.

- TH-1 support includes nutrients you would take if you had a cold virus— echinacea, astragalus, lemon balm (melissa officinalis), and maitake mushrooms.

- Th-2 support includes pine bark extract, grape seed extract, green tea extract, acai berry extract, and Pycnogenol.® These are antioxidant compounds with immune activating (pushing) properties.

Autoimmunity: If you have an autoimmune condition such as Hashimoto's hypothyroidism, stimulating immune system activity, could make your symptoms worse. Instead, use **resveratrol and curcumin** to dampen the two major inflammatory pathways in autoimmunity—TH-17 and NF-kappaB. These two products can be used in high doses. You can gradually increase their dosages until a noticeable anti-inflammatory effect is obtained. Thankfully, most flavonoids and nutritional antioxidants do not simulate the immune system, but rather, indirectly, and gently support the immune system, making them helpful in cases of autoimmunity as well.

L-Glutamine* / Glycine / Cysteine – These three amino acids are required to make the powerful antioxidant, glutathione. From a teeter-totter perspective, getting the right balance of each of these has a profound health effect in all body systems. Besides these three, selenium, cordyceps, and gotu kola can have profound effects on glutathione levels.

- L-glutamine is often used by patients with leaky gut because of its healing benefits in the small intestine. L-glutamine is transported into the cell, converted to glutamate, and readily available for intracellular glutathione synthesis.

- Glycine is needed to make important compounds, such as glutathione, creatine, and collagen. It has also been used to protect the liver from toxins and excess alcohol and to improve sleep quality and heart health.

- N-Acetyl Cysteine (NAC) is a powerful liver detoxifier being used in prescription form to treat acetaminophen overdose. It can reduce mucous build-up and is also helpful for reducing the symptoms of anxiety caused by poor chemical detoxification.

Lysine / Arginine – Lysine is often needed in high amounts in cases of liver congestion since the liver is a jailhouse for viruses. High persistent stresses in life cause a prison riot and viruses often "escape," expressing themselves in the form of cold sores, mouth ulcers, rashes, or shingles.

Lysine can help these conditions by blocking the intracellular transport of arginine, which these viruses need to replicate. People with these issues must avoid nuts and seeds, which have high levels of arginine. Lysine also aids in calcium absorption, stress reduction, and wound healing.

Arginine is a powerful vasodilator, which can ameliorate poor circulation, angina, and erectile dysfunction. It also improves heart function, kidney detoxification, and stabilizes hormones.

Branched-Chain Amino Acids (BCAAs)* — As part of an adrenaline dominance recovery program, BCAAs are often essential. The reason being, under the influence of ever-present adrenaline, a high degree of muscle burning to make fuel takes place. The primary components of this catabolic process are the three primary BCAAs—leucine, isoleucine, and valine. Taking them in supplement form provides the body with a usable source of these nutrients so that muscle breakdown is diminished.

Collagen* — Collagen is a source of easily digestible protein that is helpful for the same reasons as are the BCAAs mentioned above. Aging and adrenaline surges have a strong negative impact on collagen production and maintenance. Collagen is the most abundant protein in the body and helps give structure to our hair, skin, nails, bones, ligaments, and tendons. Thanks to collagen, we are better able to move, bend and stretch. Collagen also helps hair shine, skin glow, and nails to stay strong.

ADDITIONAL NUTRIENTS

Liver Support

- Milk thistle* seed extract
- Dandelion root extract
- Gotu kola extract
- Panax ginseng
- DL-methionine

Yeast, Bacteria and Parasite Support

- Yeast overgrowth — undecylenic acid, caprylic acid, morinda citrifolia,
- Parasites — wormwood extract, black walnut extract, olive leaf extract, garlic extract
- Bacterial overgrowth and H. Pylori – berberine, yerba mansa, oregano extract, olive leaf extract

Inflammation Support for Gut and Brain — For people with severe intestinal or brain inflammation. The flavonoids (colorful plant compounds) listed below can help.

- Gut Inflammation – lycopene, apigenin, quercetin
- Brain Inflammation, use the gut flavonoids plus luteolin, baicalein, resveratrol, rutin, catechin, curcumin

Bile support (removes toxins from the body)

- Dandelion root extract
- Milk thistle seed extract
- Ginger root
- Phosphatidylcholine
- Taurine

Leaky Gut Support

- Deglycyrrhizinated licorice
- Aloe leaf extract
- Tillandsia
- Marshmallow extract
- Gamma oryzanol
- Slippery elm bark*
- German chamomile
- Marigold flower extract
- Arabinogalactan
- Activated charcoal
- Liquid chlorophyll
- Aloe juice
- Mastic gum

Methylation Support (cellular detoxification)

- Choline
- Trimethylglycine
- MSM
- Beet root*
- Betaine HCl

Brain Support

- Acetylcholine activity — alpha-GPC, choline, huperzine A, acetyl L-carnitine, pantothenic acid

- GABA activity — valerian root, lithium orotate, passionflower extract, L-theanine, taurine, P-5-P (B6), magnesium, zinc, manganese

- Dopamine activity — mucuna pruriens, beta-phenylethylamine (PEA), blueberry extract, selenium, alpha lipoic acid, N-acetylcysteine, D, L-Phenylalanine (DLPA)an, L-tyrosine, P-5-P (B6), copper

- Serotonin Activity – L-tryptophan, 5-HTP, calcium citrate, St. John's-wort, SAMe, P-5-P (B6), niacinamide, magnesium, folic acid, B12

Heavy Metal Support – I have left this topic for last intentionally. Detoxifying heavy metals like mercury and lead can be precarious. Releasing these toxic substances too quickly can cause significant inflammatory spikes and neurological deficits that can be debilitating. Therefore, I do not recommend a heavy metal cleanse until CORE 4 balancing has begun and the *Gentle GI Diet* has been followed for at least twenty-one days. This allows time for proper gut and immune barrier healing, after which, one or more of the substances below can be used to strategically pull and eliminate heavy metals from the body.

- Alpha-lipoic acid (ALA)
- Activated charcoal
- Glutathione support
- Liver / Bile support
- Leaky Gut Support

SEVEN RULES FOR SUPPLEMENTS

Nutritional supplementation is highly effective for a variety of ailments[23] [24] [25] and consequently has led to a multi-billion-dollar vitamin industry. According to the Council for Responsible Nutrition, around 40 percent of all people in the U.S. and a majority of women over the age of 50 are taking some form of dietary supplementation.[26]

Proof of its popularity is visible in gyms, grocery stores and even gas stations, where supplements are readily available. In urban areas, stand-alone vitamin stores are commonplace, containing floor-to-ceiling displays of all the latest and greatest products.

Here is where the confusion sets in: given the number of possibilities right before their eyes, how can consumers, even knowledgeable ones, know which version of a product is right for them? Certainly, the vitamins cannot all be the same.

The best a consumer can do is to make her choice based upon quality and perhaps research. But there is more—much more. Presented below are the seven reasons why supplementation may have no beneficial effect whatsoever.

Rule #1: Is It What It Says It Is and Nothing Else?

The quality and purity of any ingested product is a chief concern for consumers and is one of the main regulatory assignments of the Food and Drug Administration. Unfortunately, what is on the label is not always what is in the package.

In a University of Maryland Pharmacy School study in 2000, only 2 of 32 different joint supplements (containing chondroitin sulfate) met the label claim for ingredients. THE STUDY REPORTED THE LESS EXPENSIVE THE SUPPLEMENT, THE LOWER THE TOTAL LEVELS OF THE NUTRIENT.[27] Unfortunately, several similar studies have been performed on a variety of different types of supplements only to find the same results.[28] [29]

Another concern with supplements is their overall quality. Despite claims of purity on the label, as a percentage, very few companies truly measure up. Poor quality means a product full of binders, fillers, and lubricants. Magnesium sterate, ascorbyl palmitate, lactose, and sodium benzoate are just a few examples. These cost-cutting and production-assisting additives can lead to poor absorption and potential allergic reactions. Beyond this, the methods of preparation and storage of raw materials is very important to avoid possible contaminants such as molds, bacteria, or heavy metals.

Rule #2: Is It What People Need with Nothing Else?

Each person is unique. This means that supplements, even ultra-pure supplements, might work for one person but not for others. Just because vitamin C is good to help the immune system, does not mean it is good in every case. In fact, depending upon the type of immune system imbalance it could instead make things worse.

Rule #3: Multi-Vitamins Are for Healthy People

Recognizing that extra nutrients are needed in the diet, a large percentage of people have become proactive, even religious, by taking multivitamins. The assumption is a once-a-day multiple-vitamin containing B-vitamins, minerals, antioxidants and the latest wild berry plucked from an isolated rock outcropping in Papua New Guinea will meet the nutritional needs of the body. If only it were that easy. For those with functional illness, just taking a multi-vitamin will probably not work. In the case of autoimmunity, it could even get worse. **Multiple vitamins are only effective for healthy people or those who are severely nutritionally deprived.**[30] The reason multivitamins are ineffective, even detrimental, has everything to do with the next rule.

Rule #4: Anything Can Be Canceled Out or Neutralized

It is not surprising to see a patient carry a large box of supplements into the office and then crash it on my desk. As soon as this happens, I know I am about to be a hero. In some cases, it is possible to take the patient off half to two-thirds of her supplements, while seeing her health improve. Most vitamin collectors are well-informed and have made wise choices based upon the latest eBlast from a respected alternative health doctor or vitamin store. Yes, everything they are taking is of good quality, and the latest research "proves" the supplements have positive health benefits. But it is a simple case of too much of a good thing becoming a bad thing.

Researchers do not conduct studies with patients taking ten or more nutrients at the same time. This would be bad science due to too many variables. Unneeded nutrients in excess will themselves tilt teeter-totters and become a cause of CORE 4 imbalances.

For example, a patient may complain about extended soreness after exercise. This is often a need for vitamin B1, which the muscles use to break down lactic acid. The same patient may complain of chronic allergies. This is often a need for vitamin B6, which is important for metabolizing histamine. So, why not give him a B-complex that has plenty of vitamin B1 and plenty of vitamin B6? Because it probably won't work. He needs vitamin B1 and vitamin B6 in isolation without interference from the rest of the family.

Vitamins teeter with vitamins, and minerals totter with minerals. Oils compete with oils, and amino acids compete with amino acids. They can all potentially cancel each other out. Finding the precise nutrient (see STEP 1) and giving that alone, without interference from others, is what makes miracles happen.

Rule #5: Everything Is on a Teeter-Totter

I hope you are beginning to see the need for the teeter-totters to be in balance. Using a multi-vitamin to raise the low side of the teeter-totter will never work since a multi-vitamin, by definition, will also contain the high or opposite nutrient as well. This means the lower nutrient will never balance out with the higher one.

Rule #6 – As the Body Changes, So Do Supplements

When I ask the patient with the shopping-bags-worth of supplements how long they have been taking their stockpile, "years" is a common answer. Just as there is no perfect food, there is no perfect supplement. Nothing should be taken for years. That is because the body is always in a state of change, adapting to life's many stresses. With changes in life, there are changes in needs.

When "filling empty buckets" with hormetic nutrients, positive changes can happen fast This means after just a few weeks some of the original buckets may start to overflow. When this occurs, it is time to slow down the dosage or stop taking that nutrient altogether. It may also mean it is time to fill up a different bucket.

Hormetic nutrients are not just *Band-Aids*—they correct problems. If a person needs the same supplements for extended periods of time and their problem is not getting fixed, then something was missed.

> **Using nutrients long-term is only necessary when they are fortifying a genetic concern or when they are needed to support an ongoing stressful situation with no immediate end in sight.**

RULE # 7 – FIXING CHRONIC PROBLEMS IS UNNATURAL

"My supplement is made from organic whole food ingredients like those found in nature." This is the argument by both patients and health professionals. On paper, these forms of supplements sound like the best things to take to restore health. Unfortunately, often they are not. Or, if they do work, they require massive doses (and great expense) and a "healing crisis" to produce results. Medicines are based on chemicals found in plants, but in an isolated form, making them much more potent than when they were combined with other ingredients in their natural state. This is a clue. **The more pure or isolated a substance, the more powerful its effect. In other words, purity equals potency.**

The more severe or chronic the problems are, the greater the nutritional deficiencies will be and the more likely it is that hormetic nutrients need to be used by themselves. Therefore, to produce powerful healing without terrible side-effects of a medicine, it is best to choose the single-use, purified, high dosage, and out-of-balance option over the general use, complex-chemical, and "naturally balanced" one. However, different hormetic nutrients **from different categories** can be used together for maximum effect. That is how I created *Core4Powder*.

These seven rules are the scientific reality of supplemental nutrition. Supplement overload is the reason many in the alternative field, who are doing things naturally, still fail to help those in need. Understanding and applying these rules equals fewer supplements, lesser cost, less burdensome lifestyle changes, quicker responses, and lasting results.

STEP 6: RESTERCISE – PAIN EQUALS NO GAIN

EXERCISE FOR AN OPTIMAL METABOLISM - INTENSE FITNESS EXERCISE TURNS ON FIGHT-OR-FLIGHT

In the same way that love covers a multitude of wrongs, exercise covers a multitude of dietary and lifestyle transgressions. No single therapy has as great an impact on the body as exercise. The blood sugar, respiratory, immune, lymphatic, digestive, musculoskeletal, energy, emotional, and every other system benefit from proper, regular exercise.[31]

Proper exercise greatly reduces total body inflammation by regulating the fight-or-flight response (which ignites everything). Additionally, as exercise burns fat, the fat cells themselves release appetite-suppressing and satiety chemicals, called lipokines.[32]

Here is a final head-scratching example: Exercise is so powerful that it not only lowers health risks, but...

active obese individuals have lower morbidity and mortality than normal weight individuals who are sedentary.[33]

This means the normal weight couch-potato who takes comfort that he or she is not "fat," is more likely to suffer from illness or die compared to his overweight, exercising neighbor. The bathroom scale is not always a good indicator of health.

This is all interesting and wonderful, but there are some critical caveats. The general rule is *a person who is healthy may use all forms of exercise, but not all exercise makes a person healthy*. Why? The wrong type of exercise perpetuates adrenaline surges making it impossible to heal adrenaline dominance. That is why I coined the term, **Restercise**: to remind patients to keep their exercise calm and slow.

Just imagine how you would feel if you were suddenly scared by a near car crash. Adrenaline would surge and disrupt your body for hours after the near miss. Intentionally spiking adrenaline through intense exercise does the same thing, igniting the whole fight-or-flight chemical cascade.

Making this mental transition is difficult for those who have spent their whole lives in the no-pain-no-gain mindset. In the past, going to the gym meant taking a spin or cardio class to "get my heart rate up." That approach will keep your body stuck in fight-or-flight. These people are in many ways fit, but most are in no way healthy.

FITNESS VS. HEALTH

When an athlete allows his body to adapt to the various stressors that he has placed upon it, the body can most certainly become fit. The fit athlete, having trained his body appropriately, is able to perform strenuous and astounding feats, yet this benefit will most likely come at the expense of other tissues and often at the expense of health itself.

On a personal note, before I ever knew anything about exercise, nutrition, and the adverse effects of stress, I was able to maintain a high degree of fitness from regular exercise. Basketball and weightlifting were an integral part of my week. If a stranger looked at me, he would think I was in good shape and healthy. Yet, with any sort of sustained stress, I would usually get sick. Other signs were also present, including chronic mucus in my throat, frequent sniffling, sneezing, achy joints from time to time, swelling in my left knee, and allergies to cats, dogs, and various foods (all of this before I was 30!). Although I was able to lift weights for two hours at a time and play basketball half of the day, I was still plagued with numerous symptoms. I may have been fit, but I was not healthy.

Most exercise programs that exclusively utilize the no-pain-no-gain approach are unintentionally producing the same problems among the public. It is not uncommon to hear of a well-known athlete having his career cut short due to nagging injuries or even by unexpected death while training. People can assume certain deficiencies of nutrients will arise when training for fitness and not for health. These deficiencies will eventually result in significant CORE 4 imbalances. This is because fitness training causes adrenaline to surge and places heavy burdens on the body's anaerobic (sugar burning) system while neglecting the more important aerobic (oxygen and fat burning) system.

THE ANAEROBIC SYSTEM

The body has two ways to make energy. One uses oxygen, the other does not. No oxygen is required with the anaerobic system. Instead, it provides quick energy by using stored blood sugar (glycogen) for fuel. This is very good so long as it is not the primary means of energy production. Bad things like excess inflammation happen when you rely on the anaerobic system long-term for daily energy.

Sprinting, fast jogging, high intensity exercise classes, and most other sports are forms of anaerobic exercise. People do these types of activities all the time. So, what is the problem?

First off, only small amounts of glycogen are available for use by the muscles at any given time. That is why weight training "sets" last only a short period before the muscles "burn out." In the presence of anxiety or fight-or-flight, anaerobic exercise forces the body to sacrifice its own muscle (catabolism) for the creation of more glucose. This requires even more adrenaline and will encourage the continuation of fight-or-flight chemistry and adrenaline dominance.

High heart rate anaerobic exercise also reinforces the body to stay in the sugar-using, fat-storing, anaerobic metabolism. Finally, too much anaerobic exercise leaves behind a great deal of inflammation leading to nagging injuries, illness, and immune system disruptions.

AEROBICS IS NOT AEROBIC

In the old days when people went to an "aerobics" class, it was for the purpose of breaking a good sweat. The movements were nonstop, and the heart rate was high. It was the equivalent intensity of today's Zumba class. Aerobic training, on the other hand, is much less intense and keeps a steady low heart rate. Examples include light jogging, easy swimming, easy biking, and a specific style of weightlifting discussed below. The aerobic system uses plenty of oxygen, which is necessary for burning fat. And of equal importance, proper aerobic exercise (Restercise) heals adrenaline dominance.

TWO TYPES OF MUSCLE FIBERS

There are two types of skeletal muscle fibers: fast and slow. Fast fibers are also called anaerobic fibers, while slow fibers are called aerobic fibers. Your genes often determine how much of each is present. Through training, an athlete can change the function of a particular fiber, making a slow fiber act like a fast fiber and vice versa. Once training has stopped, however, the cells gradually return to their previous genetically determined state.

Sprinters and bodybuilders do not have the same number of slow fibers as long-distance athletes. Instead, they have more fast fibers. All athletes, which includes everyone who exercises regularly, have certain special needs. However, it is interesting to note that athletes participating in fast fiber sports perform better if they train their slow fibers as well.

BURN FAT, NOT SUGAR

The major fuel burned when training aerobically is fat. The same amount of fat contains more than twice as much potential fuel (9 calories/gram) as do simple carbohydrates (4 calories/gram). Therefore, when engaging the aerobic system during exercise, energy expenditure is more abundant and is fat-based.

Not only should fat be the fuel of choice for energy, but it is also the one people want to get rid of in the first place.

In conclusion, low heart rate aerobic activity is the best exercise to remove the body from fight-or-flight, promote fat loss, and increase energy. The challenge is that you cannot let your heart rate get too high.

TARGET HEART RATE

The body switches from fat burning to sugar burning at a specific heart rate. Therefore, using a heart rate monitor during exercise is highly recommended. Once the heart rate exceeds a certain range, the aerobic system is disengaged, and the anaerobic system takes over. This means stored sugars—not stored fat—will become the fuel of choice. All aerobic benefit is potentially lost when training at a non-aerobic heart rate (too fast).

FINDING YOUR TARGET HEART RATE RANGE:

The following information is adapted from the book, *In Fitness and In Health,* authored by Dr. Phil Maffetone, who has successfully worked with many elite athletes to improve their aerobic capacity and overall performance. TO FIND YOUR IDEAL RANGE...

SUBTRACT YOUR **AGE** FROM THE NUMBER **180.**

NOW ADD OR SUBTRACT FROM THIS NUMBER BASED UPON THE FOLLOWING:

- **SUBTRACT 10 POINTS**—If recovering from a major illness, surgery, or taking daily medication.

- **SUBTRACT 5 POINTS**—If you have not exercised before; have exercised but have been injured or are regressing; experience frequent colds or flu or are under high stress.

- **SUBTRACT 0 POINTS**—If you have been exercising for up to two years without any real problems and have not had colds or flu more than once or twice per year.

- **ADD 5 POINTS**—If you have been exercising for more than two years without any real problems and have been making progress in your program or competitions.

THIS FINAL NUMBER IS THE UPPER END OF YOUR HEART RATE RANGE.

TO FIND THE LOWER END...

SUBTRACT 10 POINTS FROM THE UPPER NUMBER.

For example, the heart rate number for a 50-year-old-man would be 130 (180-50). But he also rarely exercises and gets the flu and/or a cold most years, so the person would need to subtract another 5 points to end up with an upper number of 125. The overall range is 10 points below the upper number or 115-125 bpm. This is his fat-burning heart rate zone. Exercising exclusively within this ten-point range will yield the greatest aerobic return and generate the highest level of fat-burning.

WHAT TO EXPECT

When first using a heart rate monitor, regular runners and those who exercise two or three times per week with no apparent difficulty are shocked by how quickly their heart rate exceeds its maximum range. Not surprisingly, these same patients showed many signs of adrenaline dominance along with nagging injuries.

They needed to slow down first to build a solid aerobic base. Those who did saw terrific results. After training in their aerobic range for 6 to 12 weeks, they were able to resume their previous running course and speed but with a much slower (healthier) heart rate.

DON'T DO TOO MUCH

The ultimate goal of training in the aerobic heart rate zone is to improve aerobic function, which means using oxygen to burn fat. A light sweat, easy breathing, and a feeling of not having done too much once exercise is finished are all good signs that training was below the maximum heart rate. Another sign is the presence of sore muscles.

Since most people have inadvertently exercised too hard, they have overtrained their fast fibers, and neglected their slow fibers. Training at a lower heart rate uses the slow (fat burning) fibers almost exclusively. Using previously unused muscle fibers makes them temporarily sore. This is good and will soon pass.

"I feel fine and can easily do another set." Don't. Building muscle is a fat-burning, oxygen using metabolism. So, keep it slow. In the first four to six weeks, resist the temptation to do more, even when enough strength and stamina are present to do so. I have watched many patients crash and burn because they ran ahead too fast. You do not want to flip on the adrenaline switch. Slow and steady wins the race.

WALK, DON'T JOG

Turning on the aerobic metabolism means working the big muscles in a slow steady fashion. The fight-or-flight response is like a thoroughbred running in the Kentucky Derby—it is an all-out sprint. Your racing days are over for now. Instead, imagine a draft horse pulling a cart.

To select your program, look to see which option below applies to you.

1. **I have not exercised in years:** You should begin with walking for 10-15 minutes three to four times a week. Over the next month or two, build up to 30 minutes five or six times a week and begin the aerobic-based weight training two or three times per week as described below.

   Note: *if you have bad knees or hips, replace walking with cycling. Use a stationary bike or find a flat area outside to ensure that you keep your heart rate in its target range.*

2. **I exercise semi-regularly:** You may begin aerobic-based weight training up to three times per week. Also, continue to do a "cardio" workout at least twice a week within your heart rate range. Do the *Maximum Aerobic Function Test* every three weeks to make sure you are progressing.

3. **I exercise regularly:** In your case, follow the *Restercise* weight-lifting approach. But you are free to do additional sets so long as you are keeping your heart rate in its proper range.

THE MAXIMUM AEROBIC FUNCTION TEST (MAF)

It is always a good idea to monitor exercise progress. After a few weeks of heart rate training positive signs will be present such as feeling better, not being as tired, having more energy, gaining resistance to sickness, improved sleep patterns, and more. These subjective findings are important, but a maximum aerobic function test (MAF) to check for objective changes is critical as well.

TWO WAYS TO DO THE MAF TEST – TIME OR DISTANCE?

To do an MAF test, choose a **DISTANCE** such as 4 to 8 times around the local high school track. Walk the entire distance while within your target heart rate range, speeding up or slowing down as necessary. Once the distance is completed, record the time.

After two or three weeks, repeat the MAF test. Be sure that the conditions are similar for each test. The results from a calm still day may be different than those from a wet and windy day. If, after the next MAF test, you can cover the same distance in less time while staying within the target heart rate range, then the aerobic system is improving.

The opposite can be done as well. Choose a specific amount of **TIME** to perform an exercise and measure the total distance. Progress means being able to go further on a subsequent test within the same amount of time. These tests are important emotionally because they quantitatively demonstrate progress, which encourages continued exercise.

PERFORM THE MAF TEST EVERY THREE OR FOUR WEEKS.

Most will find that they improve rather quickly, and that they need to progress from walking to fast walking or a slow jog to not fall below their heart rate range.

If improvement has not occurred, other variables should be considered like sickness, additional stress, inadequate rest, too many bad foods, etc. If so, these must be addressed/resolved for progress to resume.

AEROBIC-BASED WEIGHT TRAINING

Because of CORE 4 imbalances the body has been trained to keep the fight-or-flight response turned on. Therefore, the entire oxygen-using, fat-burning, aerobic system needs to be reestablished and the anaerobic, non-oxygen system needs to be shut off.

Weightlifting becomes the exercise of choice to accomplish this with some very specific caveats.

After the warmup, the remainder of the workout should be **no more than thirty minutes,** with as much rest between sets as needed to allow for the heart rate to return to within 10 points of its resting level.

In the beginning, **only the big muscles groups are worked, for only one set per group.** More sets and various exercises can be added after several weeks.

An example may look like this:

Warm up for 5-10 minutes with some light stretching and/or walking.

1. Pull downs (latissimus) – 12-15 reps (1 min)
   3 to 4-minute rest

2. Chest press (pectoralis) – 12-15 reps (1 min)
   3 to 4-minute rest

3. Dumbbell curls (biceps) – 12-15 reps (1 min)
   3 to 4-minute rest

4. Arm extensions (triceps) – 12-15 reps (1 min)
   3 to 4-minute rest

5. Leg extensions (quadriceps) – 12-15 reps (1 min)
   3 to 4-minute rest

6. Leg curls (hamstrings) – 12-15 reps (1 min)
   3 to 4-minute rest

Total time 25-30 minutes

The body's entire big muscle system has been asked to perform, but not for an extended duration. The moderate weight will ensure that all the muscle fibers of the big muscle group are recruited to around 80% of their capacity. This "all fibers in" approach "drains" adrenaline, "burns" fatty acids in the blood, and stimulates muscle fiber growth.

With consistency of training in this manner, the body is re-programmed to switch off the reflexive adrenaline response and is induced to build muscle in preparation for the future short and heavy workloads it now "expects" to come.

RESTERCISE FOR 4 TO 6 WEEKS

Restercise as restorative training is highly effective so long as the total exercise time is SHORT FOR THE FIRST FOUR TO SIX WEEKS. Additional exercises or exercising without enough rest will again turn on adrenaline to manage what the body now perceives to be a survival response.

As the body transforms and reprograms itself based on this training, it will soon demonstrate the benefits through increased strength and a quicker heart rate recovery between sets. AT THIS POINT, MORE SETS AND MORE TIME CAN BE ADDED IN A STEADY, METHODICAL WAY.

WHEN IS THE BEST TIME TO EXERCISE?

Without some fuel in the tissues from food, the body uses its stored glucose (glycogen) and will burn up muscle tissue to make more glucose if needed. Those who like to exercise first thing in the morning are especially prone to this problem.

All night you have gone without food, using up most of your stored sugar and dipping into your reserves. This may sound good for fat loss, but there is a catch.

Speeding up the heart or overly exerting the muscles in a low sugar state will trigger adrenaline surges and sabotage long-term benefits. Having a small amount of a protein/fat/carb "snack" before beginning your early morning routine is essential. Better yet, exercise later in the day after a meal or two.

When beginning *Restercise* to heal adrenaline dominance and build your aerobic base, exercise should be either two hours after breakfast or an hour before dinner.

It is best not to exercise after dinner because you should be training your body and mind to CALM DOWN IN THE EVENINGS. Going to the gym and working out under the artificial lights while jamming to your favorite upbeat tunes does the opposite.

The one exception would be a stretching routine at home in a dimmed light setting. Doing this for twenty minutes or less could help the wind-down process.

WARMING UP AND STRETCHING

Warming up and stretching are essential, but they are not the same thing. Warming up should always happen first and is as simple as a slow easy walk for 10 minutes. It is necessary to prepare the body for exercise and to prevent injury. Warming up also begins the fat-burning process by promoting the release of free-floating fatty acids, the desired energy source.

Up to 80 percent of the blood in the organs will be transferred to the muscles during exercise. Warming up prior to intense exercise allows this fluid transfer to happen gradually. This is important for another reason. Exercise generates vast quantities of metabolic waste products. Warming up ensures that a sufficient amount of blood is circulating prior to exercise, so these by-products can be shuttled to the liver for detoxification and elimination.

After the brief warm-up period, stretching may be performed. The added circulation from the warm-up period allows for greater elasticity and flexibility of the tissues during a stretch, decreasing the chance for injury. A person should not stretch through the point of pain and should not bounce when stretching. Stretching beyond the normal range of motion may temporarily increase flexibility, but it also leads to micro injury.

COOLING DOWN

The cool-down is just as important as the warm-up. Cooling down allows a gentle return of the blood to the various organs. Stopping suddenly after exercise causes a rapid rush of blood into the organs, bringing with it an abundance of exercise-induced waste products.

Since most blood is stored within the organs during times of inactivity, without a cool down, chemical waste products may amass. The potential toxic buildup, if severe enough, could mean most of the aerobic benefits from the exercise are lost. At the end of the walk/jog, simply reduce the exercise pace gradually until the heart rate is about 10 - 20 beats above the resting heart rate. This process is all that is needed and should only take about 10 minutes.

EXERCISE AND YOUR JOINTS

Chiropractors have made their living aiding the joints (especially the 24 vertebral segments of the spine) by restoring full movement throughout their designed physiologic range.

The beneficial results of regular adjustments, such as pain relief and increased flexibility, have been experienced by millions. But there is much more to this story.

There 360 joints made up from the body's 206 bones. Joints are what allow for movement as muscles contract and relax. Movement has obvious benefits and some, related to the nervous system and genetics, that are just now being understood.

The connection between the nervous system and the genes is the reason the chiropractic adjustment has a profound impact on health—one that goes well beyond pain reduction and increased motion.

Adjustments are one of the primary therapies I use to aid in emotional stress reduction, allergy elimination, immune system balance, and detoxification.

Why? Turns out, these positive outcomes are all linked to the proper motion of the joints and the profound neurological benefit their motion brings. Move it, or lose it, is not just a slogan.

Motion is foundational to health.

MOVE IT OR LOSE IT

The nervous system, that marvelous transmitter of electrical and chemical messages which governs the majority of bodily functions, is intimately connected to, supported, and enhanced by, feedback from the joints.

The relationship between the nervous system and the joints is so interdependent that reduced feedback from a lack of motion will interfere with the proper expression of our genes, what is called protein transcription.[34] This is not good at all.

Since genetics are the human body's intrinsic defense system, health is not possible without their appropriate expression.

Let me put that another way...

IF YOU DO NOT MOVE YOUR BODY THROUGH ALL ITS DESIGNED RANGES OF MOTION, AND DO SO ON A REGULAR BASIS, YOU GREATLY INCREASE YOUR CHANCES OF INCURRING AN INCONVENIENT CONDITION, ILLNESS, OR DISEASE.

So, get busy Restercising!

STEP 7: RESTORE SLEEP & BIORHYTHMS

RESTORE SLEEP, BALANCE BIORHYTHMS, AND RETRAIN THE BRAIN TO RELAX
AGAIN, ALL WITH A PROPER NIGHTTIME ROUTINE

SLEEP AND EXERCISE

Sleep and exercise are linked via certain hormones in a balanced interrelationship that must be carefully maintained. With proper sleep, exercise becomes the means for increased strength, fitness, and detoxification. With proper exercise, sleep is more restful and restorative. Finally, sleep and exercise working together are the power supply for the body's internal clocks and biorhythms.

Sleep is a time of neurological detoxification and tissue repair. Without sleep, concentration lessens, response slows, and the pathways for learning, creating, and recalling memories do not fully form. This is true mostly because the hormones in your brain, called neurotransmitters, are hindered from returning to their proper levels. The most important hormone for healing and restoration is human growth hormone.

Human growth hormone (HGH) is a complex protein produced by the pituitary gland in the brain and is an essential part of the body's endocrine (hormonal) system. It promotes a healthy metabolism, enhances physical performance, and may even increase longevity. **Up to 75% of HGH is released by the brain into the bloodstream during sleep.** Most of the remaining HGH is released during exercise. This is how the teeter-totter balance between sleep and exercise is inseparably linked.

SLEEP RESETS OUR CIRCADIAN RHYTHM

Circadian rhythms are biological processes that every plant, animal, and human, exhibits over the course of a day. These rhythms are governed by a master clock located in the brain and by trillions of other clocks found inside every cell of your body.

Thousands of genes, which influence all aspects of health, are turned on or off by these cellular clocks at different times of the day or night. When sleep is disrupted and the daily rhythms are disturbed for even as little as a day or two, our clocks cannot send out the right messages to these genes, and the body and mind begin to slip out of balance. [35]

CLOCKS AND RHYTHMS

Perhaps the two most studied and well-recognized human cycles are the daily and monthly cycles. The daily cycle, called the circadian rhythm, governs the sleep and wake cycle, body temperature, metabolism, and the release of hormones, while the monthly cycle, called the menstrual cycle, governs the monthly rhythm of female hormones.

If any chemical substances could be said to oversee the inward cycles, it would be hormones. Interaction between these powerful protein molecules create *biorhythms*.

Disruptions of the normal physiological ebb and flow are a sign that adrenaline dominance is already underway and that functional illness and future disease are likely such as: anxiety and depression, [36] poor memory, [37] increased breast cancer rates in women, [38] increased cardiovascular disease, [39] hypoglycemia, and metabolic syndrome. [40]

STOP THE LIGHT AT NIGHT!

Specialized cells in the retinas of your eyes process light and tell the brain whether it is day or night. So do receptors in your skin. However, the sleep-wake cycle is easily altered by exposure to prolonged artificial light such as when staying up late watching television, working on the computer, working the night shift, or even just by crossing several time zones.

Deep, restful sleep is dependent upon several factors, but a critical one is the rhythm between two hormones: cortisol and melatonin. Cortisol must be at high levels in the morning and at low levels at night. Melatonin is just the opposite. It increases at night when things get dark.

The absence of light causes the pineal gland in the brain to become active, encouraging additional melatonin production. **Simply turning the lights down to low levels and intentionally going to sleep before 10 p.m. can help a great deal.**

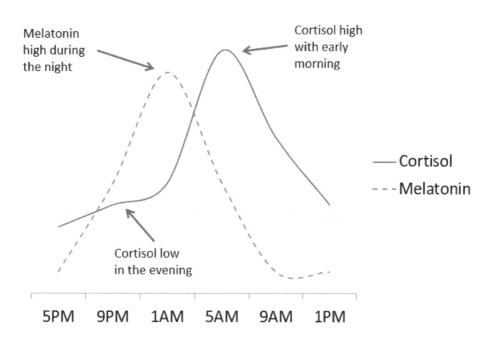

Figure 1: Normal Circadian Rhythm

Those with functional imbalances do not have the above normal pattern. This means the levels of cortisol are often the inverse of what they should be, while melatonin never reaches a level sufficient for deep sleep. Signs related to disrupted circadian rhythms include the inability to fall asleep or stay asleep, difficulty waking up in the morning, not feeling rested after sleep, a drop in energy between 4 and 7 p.m., and headaches in the daytime (a diurnal pattern).

Abnormal Circadian Rhythm

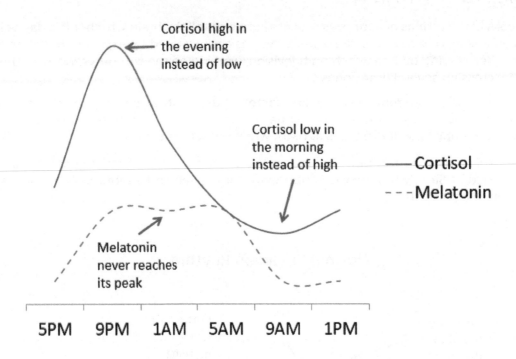

Figure 2: Abnormal Circadian Rhythm

THE TWELVE-HOUR CYCLE

The *50 FIX Plan* is designed to synchronize the body into its daily circadian rhythm. This means starting your day at sunrise and winding down in the evening. A twelve-hour schedule of 6 or 7 a.m. to 6 or 7 p.m. is ideal. **During this time, you will have done your daily work, had your three blood-sugar-balancing meals, been in the sun for at least fifteen minutes, and have completed your** *Restercise.* The final three to four hours of the day (hours 13 through 16) should be in a low-light, calming atmosphere that culminates in sleep no more than three hours after your last meal.

Sample Daily Schedule:

6:15 a.m. — wake up

7:15 a.m. — breakfast

8 a.m. to 12:30 p.m. — work

12:30 p.m. — lunch (a good time for some sunlight)

1:30 to 5 p.m. – work

5:45 p.m. — exercise

6:45 p.m. — dinner (or 6 p.m. on non-exercise days)

9:30 p.m. — sleep

On exercise days, when the schedule is stretched for an extra hour (dinner at 6:45 p.m. instead of 6 p.m.) there are still over two, and less than three and a half, hours before going to bed. This allows ample time for food to digest. Going to bed no longer than three hours after your dinner helps to keep blood sugar more stable throughout the night. Going to bed too soon leads to upset digestion and poor liver detoxification.

HOW MUCH SLEEP IS ENOUGH?

Babies initially sleep as much as 16 to 18 hours per day, which is likely related to brain and body development (especially the brain). School-age children and teens on average need about 9.5 hours of sleep per night. People who consistently sleep too little are more likely to die early than those who get the full 7 hours of sleep each night. Similarly, people who sleep as much as 10 to 11 hours are also likely to live shorter lives. Most people who had an ideal weight-to-height ratio, nearly all slept 7 hours a night..[41]

I ONLY NEED 3 OR 4 HOURS OF SLEEP?

Some adults will say that they only need three or four hours of sleep per night. They are gamblers, risking their hard-earned health because of a lucky streak. Yes, they can do it for a time, maybe even years, but not allowing the nervous system to rest and enjoy the healing benefits of growth hormone will take its toll. The bottom line is that too much or too little sleep can be detrimental. [42]

Recovering from adrenaline dominance is not possible without sleep, but **sleep is nearly impossible when the fight-or-flight response is raging.** That is why an all-hands-on-deck approach is required to get the ship sailing straight again. This is what the *50 FIX Plan* is designed to do. Here are some practical tips for getting and staying asleep:

SLEEP TIPS

- **WALK IN THE LIGHT** — Regular sunlight exposure is critical for health. Sunlight establishes your circadian "clock" by regulating levels of serotonin and melatonin—an anti-cancer hormone. The UV light from early and mid-day sun signals the body to make vitamin D, whereas the infrared light that comes later in the day is anti-inflammatory. Sunlight also boosts mood, strengthens the immune system, and even kills bacteria. Get at least 30 minutes of sun exposure on your skin each day.

- **YOU ARE NOT A NIGHT OWL** — The brain clock synchronizes with the morning light and starts counting the hours we are awake. For most people, after being up for twelve hours, the brain begins to gently nudge us into a more relaxed state so that soon we can go to sleep. [43] **If you tend to have more energy at night it is because your entire body clock is out of rhythm from CORE 4 imbalances.** You need to create a new sleep schedule. Do everything listed below.

- **SET A SCHEDULE** – Go to bed and wake up at the same time each day. The body benefits greatly from routine (it also needs variety, but that comes later after some balancing in the CORE 4 and your nutritional reserves have been built up). As stated earlier, I recommend a twelve-hour daily cycle wherein the three meals of the day are eaten, and exercise has taken place. Then sleep should be no later than three (perhaps four) hours after the last meal. This is to make sure there is plenty of stored blood sugar in the muscles and liver to be used by the brain during sleep. Going to sleep more than four hours after eating can trigger an adrenaline surge during the night, disrupting sleep and destabilizing blood sugar levels.

- **AVOID CAFFEINE, NICOTINE, AND ALCOHOL BEFORE BED** — There are some people who can drink a pot of coffee and fall asleep a few minutes later. These folks have low dopamine levels and are stuck in chronic fight-or-flight. For the rest of you, caffeine at dinner or before bed will keep adrenaline surges pumping resulting in significant negative effects on sleep.

- **RELAX BEFORE BED** – Try a warm bath, reading, or another relaxing routine. Your body will start to come down and your mind calm down when signaled to do so by your daily habits.

- **CREATE A ROOM FOR SLEEP** – Avoid bright lights and loud sounds and keep the room at a comfortable temperature. Most importantly, do not watch TV or have a computer in your bedroom. This is a big deal. People who watch television right up until the moment they go to sleep have greatly stressed their body clock and confused their pineal gland (the light awareness gland). Likewise, having the TV on every moment, even playing in the background with guests in the house, indicates a deficiency of inner quiet and an ever-present state of adrenaline dominance. Simply doing your daily tasks in a state of quiet, absent of needless background noise, will help to reprogram the fight-or-flight response.

- **DON'T LIE IN BED AWAKE** — If you cannot get to sleep, try reading or listening to acoustic music until you feel tired. Sleep research is showing that going to bed tired and for the purpose of sleep (not watching TV or browsing social media) is a strong trigger for brain relaxation and sleep-hormone release. Many people never get tired because they never make their bodies tired during the day with exercise.

- **GET TIRED** —As discussed in STEP 6: RESTERCISE, exercise is one of the greatest sleep aides if done properly and at the right time. The right time is usually later in the day, but not after 8 p.m. Just before dinner works well. Early morning workouts are often too excitatory and can spike adrenaline. There is also a shortage of glycogen because it has been used for fuel all night. This makes it easy to over-exercise in the morning and reignite the fight-or-flight response.

- **COUNT YOUR BLESSINGS** — So many people cannot stop their minds from thinking about the day's activities. Think instead about all the good things in your life—what you have, who you know, who you love, and who loves you, etc. Often the worries of tomorrow fade away when we remember the blessings of today.

- **PRACTICE TENSION RELEASE** — As you are lying in bed, think about whatever area of your body is holding tension. Then, while concentrating on it, breathe in slowly and deeply and when you exhale, imagine the tension leaving the tissues. Repeat these steps until the tension is gone. Now, do this for any other areas you discover. The mind has a powerful ability to remove pain and tension when put to proper use.

STEP 8: REPLACE TRAPPED EMOTIONS

USE A POWERFUL NEUROLOGICAL TECHNIQUE TO REMOVE TRAPPED CIRCULATING EMOTIONS AND REPLACE THEM WITH CALMING, CONSTRUCTIVE THOUGHTS

Psychoneuroimmunology is a field of study that recognizes the impact of emotions on physical health. Unresolved emotions such as grief, anxiety, and anger, direct human action more than people realize, doing so on an unconscious level and to the detriment of their own health. For instance, my patients who use continuous glucose monitors have shown me how an emotionally distressing experience kept their blood sugar levels elevated in the danger zone for two or three days! Negative emotions are also one of the greatest epigenetic factors turning "on" or "off" good and bad genes. This is all bad. But zero negative emotion is not always good.

NAVIGATING POSITIVE AND NEGATIVE EMOTIONS

Positive emotions usually get all the credit when people "get motivated" and change direction leading to great personal accomplishment. But negative emotions can produce the same results. Being called "fat," "slow," "ugly," "dumb," or any other derogatory word may create a downward spiral of self-pity, unproductive thoughts, and unhealthy behaviors. In another, negative emotions may be the catalyst to effort, persistence, healthy habits, and an overcoming spirit. Most of history's heroes were created because of negative emotions and experiences. Negative emotions, like inflammation, have a significant role to play. We just don't want too much of either.

Likewise, positive emotions are not always good. The parent who showers with "love" but fails to restrain or correct his child immediately, is likely to end up with a selfish little monster. Societies who fail to enforce boundaries and pass out entitlements by political reflex end up with selfish citizens. These both are a result of too much positive emotion. It is about balance.

No one is born an emotional boxing champion. It is a skill acquired by sparing with positive and negative feelings in the ring of life. Withstanding the emotional body blows and fighting back with a flurry of counterpunches is a sign of good mental health. If this doesn't happen, a third method for dealing with lingering emotions inevitably occurs leading to functional illness and the creation of a neuro-emotional complex.

THE NEURO-EMOTIONAL COMPLEX

When a past event or current circumstance is overwhelming or "too much to deal with," a neurological coping mechanism initiates in the mind resulting in a Neuro-Emotional Complex (NEC). An NEC is essentially a quarantine emotion held in place until the body has the capacity to heal and move beyond it. Correction can and does happen naturally and unconsciously. However, oftentimes direct intervention is required.

The origins of some NECs are obvious — the child who was molested, the anxiety-filled teenager who didn't fit in, a toxic relationship, inescapable traumatic circumstances, etc. NECs can also develop from the anxiety of repeated lesser events. In either case, once an NEC is established, imbalances in the CORE 4 are inescapable.

Trapped unconscious emotions are like water coursing through eroded rock. The negative emotional pathways pour forth in only one direction, manifesting as one or more functional illnesses. Retraining the brain through thoughts, therapies, and actions, carves a new beneficial route that replaces the negative emotion with a positive one and removes the NEC.

TAPPING AND BREATHING

Therapies such as Emotional Freedom Technique,[44] Neuro Emotional Therapy,[45] and Eye Movement Desensitization and Reprocessing (EMDR), use recall and repatterning to remove and replace trapped negative emotions.

The technique taught below does the same thing by targeting 14 Primary Energetic Points (PEPs), each with a strong connection to both a brain neurotransmitter and an emotion. Tapping these points and breathing slowly with a steady rate, while thinking of the negative emotion at the same time, is a profound way to remove NECs and calm momentary anxieties.

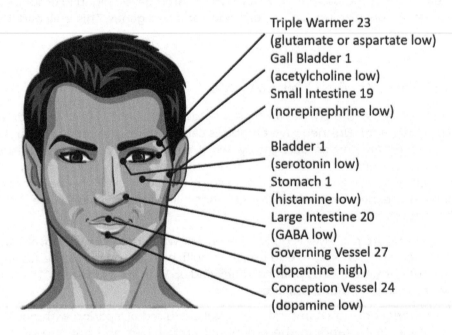

Triple Warmer 23
(glutamate or aspartate low)
Gall Bladder 1
(acetylcholine low)
Small Intestine 19
(norepinephrine low)

Bladder 1
(serotonin low)
Stomach 1
(histamine low)
Large Intestine 20
(GABA low)
Governing Vessel 27
(dopamine high)
Conception Vessel 24
(dopamine low)

Primary Energetic Point	Emotion
Triple Warmer 23	Panic / Trapped
Gall Bladder 1	Guilt / Blame / Judgmental
Bladder 1	Shame / Humiliation
Stomach 1	ANXIETY / Lethargic
Large Intestine 20	Apathy / Despair
Small Intestine 19	Indecisive / Laziness
Governing Vessel 27	Lust / Desire
Conception Vessel 24	Grief / Regret

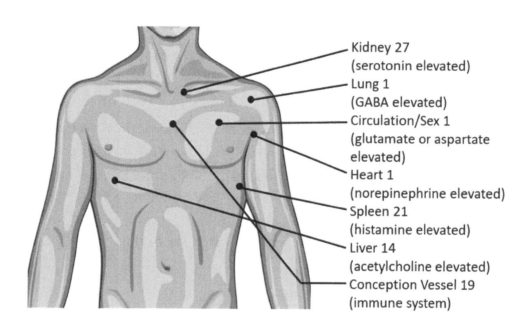

Kidney 27
(serotonin elevated)
Lung 1
(GABA elevated)
Circulation/Sex 1
(glutamate or aspartate
elevated)
Heart 1
(norepinephrine elevated)
Spleen 21
(histamine elevated)
Liver 14
(acetylcholine elevated)
Conception Vessel 19
(immune system)

Primary Energetic Point	Emotion
Kidney 27	**ANXIETY** / Fear
Lung 1	Anger / Hate
Circulation/Sex 1	Manic / Bewilderment
Heart 1	Tension / Irritation
Spleen 21	Agitation / **OVERWHELMED**
Liver 14	Anger / Pride / Scorn
Conception Vessel 19	**IMMUNE WEAKNESS**

STEPS TO CLEAR THE NEC

1. Find the PEP on the chart above related to your emotion (for ANXIETY use Stomach 1 on the front of the cheeks).

2. Rate your current emotion/circumstance (i.e., anxiety, fear, anger, etc.) on a scale of 1-10 (10 is worst).

3. While thinking of any specific details related to the emotion/circumstance, start tapping the NEC point at a rate of 2 taps per second for 30 seconds.

4. For the next 30 seconds, while still tapping, say out loud one or all the following or something similar:

    a. "I can let go of this emotion/circumstance because I have not been given a spirit of fear, but of power and a sound mind."

    b. "I expel my emotion/circumstance and replace it with peace and calm."

    c. "I have taken responsibility for my part in this emotion/circumstance and am now free."

5. Add in the eyes for deeper emotional release. Look in different directions throughout the tapping process. With eyes closed, hold one position for 5 seconds before moving to the next. Examples:

    a. Up and right (5 seconds) to down and left (5 seconds)

    b. Up and left (5 seconds) to down and right (5 seconds)

    c. Up (5 seconds) to down (5 seconds) and back up

    d. Repeat each of these steps

6. Finally, to help balance the entire electrical system, tap each of the following additional points for 20-30 seconds:

    a. **Kidney 27** (at the start of the collarbones)

    b. **Spleen 21** (three inches below the armpits – tap one at a time or rub both at the same time (monkey rub))

    c. **GV20** (top of the head)

    d. **CV24** (bottom of the lip)

7. Now re-rate your anxiety now on a scale of 1-10. There should be a significant decrease. If not, repeat this entire process until there is a 50% improvement or better.

STEP 9: RELOCATE, TAKE VITAMIN "NO"

DAILY VITAMIN "NO" IS ESSENTIAL TO ESCAPE BUSYNESS, AVOID HIGH STRESS SITUATIONS, AND TO PREVENT HEALTH SETBACKS

People are far too busy. 70% of parents are too busy to read to their children at night. Nearly 50% of Americans say that they regularly lie awake at night because of stress, and 33% of Americans are living with extreme stress daily.[46] "Busy" is now the new default state.

I have chosen the topic of busyness because many emotions are at work to make it so. What's more, how to reduce busyness is one of the most common discussions I have with my patients since it is directly related to adrenaline surges and CORE 4 imbalances. Said another way, their restless emotions are making them sick.

Busyness is not always a bad thing. In fact, it is a likely thing when attempting to develop oneself, overcome unwanted circumstances, achieve a higher socio-economic status, or when raising children. Busyness however, for survival, duty, love, service, or in the pursuit of truth is a good thing. The problem arises when essential busyness has stacked on it additional busyness for non-essential reasons. This is the scenario most find themselves in, but it should not go on forever. There are simply too many physical and emotional costs.

DECODING BUSYNESS

Human beings are highly motivated by pleasure, power, and praise. Busyness most certainly contains these components. Sadly, the contentment experienced from achieving any of them does not last long and does not put an end to busyness.

Most people achieve plenty in life – make the team, graduate school, get a degree, get a job, get married, buy a house, etc. So, discontentment should have been calmed. But very often, it is not – get a better job, get a bigger house, a nicer car, a new spouse. The mind has become restless; the heart is not satisfied. Desire fulfilled has only led to greater desire.

When I was a young man, my stepfather retired early from his law practice because the daily stress was literally killing him. One of his comments years later was that he missed the "pats on the back" and "at-a-boy's" that came from helping a client get clear of a legal jam. Which begs the question, how much of what we do in our daily lives is for the praise of others? How often do we perform, look good, and act for people just to "keep up with the Jones'?"

It appears that power, pleasure, and praise are so gratifying that we will pursue and cling to them indefinitely unless a life-altering health crisis or other emergency compels us to change direction and separate ourselves. A universal self-deception has taken place.

How is our attachment to power, pleasure, or praise a means of self-deception? Because you can't know everything, you can't do everything, you can't have everything, you can't be everywhere, and you don't live forever. Life goes fast, your material body is limited, and death is certain. This is humbling, or at least it should be. Only those with inexhaustible pride continue to seek power and praise indefinitely and believe they can attain it. They can't. Death sees to it.

Author of the book, *The Busy Trap*, Tim Kreider wrote in a NY Times editorial:

> *"It's almost always people whose lamented busyness is purely self-imposed: work and obligations they've taken on voluntarily, classes and activities they've "encouraged" their kids to participate in. They're busy because of their own ambition or drive or anxiety, because they're addicted to busyness and dread what they might have to face in its absence....*
>
> *Almost everyone I know is busy. They feel anxious and guilty when they aren't either working or doing something to promote their work. They schedule in time with friends the way students with 4.0 G.P.A.'s make sure to sign up for community service because it looks good on their college applications."* [47]

Decoding busyness further reveals that the pursuits of many are in truth, sophisticated social maneuvers to compensate for an underlying anxiety, insecurity, dissatisfaction, or discontentment within. In other words, it is a lack of peace. This is the type of busyness I see at work in most of my patients. It is the genesis of the anxiety component and a common place where adrenaline surges are ignited.

COMMUNITY ACCEPTANCE

We humans organize ourselves into whichever social groups support, accept, empower, and give us praise. This is natural and necessary because it is hard-wired into our being. We are meant to be in community.

A group or community brings with it a "benefit-of-the-doubt" that quickly forgives minor mistakes and overlooks the clumsy and awkward stages of social and personal development. A good community stabilizes the soul.

For young people, the family has traditionally been the first and greatest community. Now, much of the essential graciousness its permanent attachments provided has been replaced with less devoted, more fluid social arrangements at school, work, and on teams, making emotional stability more tenuous.

Those with a supportive group of friends who can guide them through the difficult stages of adolescence have a great advantage. However, a myriad of inner anxieties are present and the daily pursuits have not stopped. The group that sustained them through an initial stressful period may prove inadequate for the next, and so will be replaced by another community more able to support the desires of the moment.

Even an unpredictable group such as a street gang can be a desirable community. A gang provides both praise and power. It will offer power through strength in numbers and praise through dedication and loyalty. The fact that young men and women are willing to subject themselves to strict rules and severe consequences for breaking those rules, all for the sake of a community and the internal and external protection it provides, is another example of how powerful this inner drive for acceptance truly is.

As I hear about parents running to and fro, shuttling their children between athletic games, cheerleading competitions, dance camps, speech debates, and a hundred other activities, I know they are motivated for altruistic reasons, but are equally being internally pushed by many of the reasons given above.

Parents are rightly concerned for the future of their children and are willing to sacrifice their personal time to create potential opportunities for them. But their efforts may backfire. Unknowingly, moms and dads are training a new generation to believe that the way grown-ups manage their anxieties is to do more, get more, accomplish more, or achieve more.

The young adults who have respect for their parents will begin to mimic this adult behavior. The number of young people I see in my office with full blown anxiety, directly related to overachieving in sports and academics, is high and heartbreaking. Worse, however, are the ones who go the opposite direction. Seeing the strain and exhaustion on the faces of their parents, they reason to themselves, "If that is what raising kids is all about, I won't have any." Adolescents, whose bond with their parents was broken, having lost respect for them long ago, often take a path of more immediate gratification and/or self-destructive behavior. Both of which signal that the life approach presented to them by their parents was either unwanted or was unattainable. They sought another way.

COMMUNITY REJECTION

When I originally wrote this section, yet another school shooting had taken place in Colorado where I practice. This time the shooting was at one of the country's leading S.T.E.M. schools. The week prior, in India, twenty-one children committed suicide on the same day because their test scores were not high enough to satisfy the expectations of their family or community.

The media is quick to blame these tragedies on the external. Were they due to socio-economic factors? In India, perhaps, to an extent. But not likely in Colorado. The school is in Douglas County, one of the richest per capita counties in the country. The children who attend this school are selected based on higher-than-average academic ability, so their future opportunities were likely greater as well. Status and future potential, it seems, were not enough to stop extreme violence.

What is common between the two atrocities is the rejection by a community and of a community. In India, not achieving at the highest level meant remaining in a community while deemed a failure. In Colorado, the two perpetrators openly expressed their hatred for their society and its traditional norms, and doubtless, felt rejected by those norms. The pain and rage in both situations were so great, that ultimate violence was willingly undertaken toward oneself and others, respectively. THE POWER OF AN ACCEPTING COMMUNITY CANNOT BE UNDERSTATED.

Therapists have seen great success working with troubled teenagers in a wilderness setting. Some of the key strategies used to increase emotional health and stability include the following:

1. A COMMUNITY was essential to survive in the wilderness, which helped teach new communication skills and relationship skills.

2. The focus was on the basics, such as securing food and shelter, which provided PURPOSE AND MEANING.

3. Accomplishment of critical tasks established lasting SELF-CONFIDENCE.

4. Skill development led to a discovery of talents and social reward through the desire to be ACCEPTED/NEEDED. Being strongly needed is also the opposite of condemnation or rejection—two common reasons for emotional distress.

5. DAILY EXERCISE kept the body strong and functioning.

6. EATING HEALTHY meals provided replenishment of lost nutrients.

7. Eating together provided additional EMOTIONAL SATISFACTION in a community setting.

8. Keeping a REGULAR SLEEP SCHEDULE maintained proper circadian rhythms and neurological restoration.

9. Finally, the wilderness experience offered a reprieve from the EXTERNAL PRESSURES of life in a fast-paced society and the unintended pressures from school, family, and social circles that often manifest despite their overall stabilizing effects.

TWENTY SUGGESTIONS FOR BUSYNESS

1. **TAKE "VITAMIN-NO!"** — Own the idea that health is not possible without adequate physical and mental rest. Adequate is likely a lot more than you are getting now. You must say, "NO" to busyness and many good and fun things. It is your duty as the one in charge of YOU. It is necessary to break vicious stress cycles and stop adrenaline dominance.

2. **CHOOSE A LIKE-MINDED COMMUNITY** — Doing life in the wrong community is a tragedy waiting to happen. The right community will be an integral part of the peace your soul requires. However, do not just assume that your community is healthy and complete. Test THEIR BELIEFS and see if they be so.

3. **STOP TRYING SO HARD TO BE LIKED** — It is true, friendship takes work. But we all know you can't please everyone. Be selective. Choose to be around people who make you better and want the best for you. You will know them. They are the ones who tell you the truth even when it hurts, stick around in tough times, and are willing to forgive your mistakes.

4. **BE FORTIFIED** — Entropy is the universal law of decay. Doing nothing to support yourself means fight-or-flight worsens and health devolves. Conquering busyness, like anything worth doing, requires putting energy into the system. Fortify your mind and body now so that you can be strong and courageous in time of need.

5. **BE A THINKER** — Far too many people live by their emotions exclusively. Emotions are a blessing, but you also have a head, not just a heart. Think about the other side. Test YOUR BELIEFS to see if they are true. All of them. The second greatest power in the universe is the power of self-deception. Because of Madison Avenue and the media, not much in this world is as it seems. As the great philosopher Apollo Creed once said, "Be a thinker, not a stinker."

6. **LIVE TODAY LIKE YOU WOULD DIE TOMORROW** — If you knew you were going to die tomorrow, you would probably not fuss about the undone chores, or watch hours of television, or listen to gossip on social media. If you had children, you would hold them, call them, tell them you loved them, forgive them, and ask for their forgiveness. If they lived across town, you wouldn't care about looking your best, you would just put on a hat and go. On your way, you would ignore the driver who cut you off, and give fifty bucks to the homeless man at the red light. Death helps us know what is important and what to do.

7. **MAKE MARGIN A PRIORITY** — Ask yourself hard "what if" questions: What if my child got really sick? What if I was injured and couldn't work? How would you rearrange your life to be prepared for those scenarios? Maybe you need to invest more? Maybe you need to do less?

8. **DO RIGHT** — Everyone has a gripe, a right, a claim. Stop caring so much about your rights and start doing what is right—for you, and for others.

9. **DON'T BE A LONER** — People today sense that they are stuck on the hamster wheel and want to get off. Worse, they want to check out of society altogether and become a hermit. That may sound nice, but many hermits turn into selfish and self-righteous people. They live in isolation because they do not want their ideas challenged and because no one is worth their time. Everyone is worth your time. Give them some. Just don't let them have all of it.

10. **BE ALONE** — This world is constantly drawing you into busyness and discontentment. The right community will help you stay on the contentment path, but you will often need to go it alone.

Taking time for yourself to rest and recharge the mind is essential. Perhaps a hike, reading a book, or sitting in the park is balancing for you? Exercising does it for me, especially if I am getting grumpy.

11. **BE SACRED** — You are a created being, made in God's image. So is everyone else. Treat them that way. Treat yourself that way. If you have messed up, seek forgiveness from God and from others and then move on. You aren't perfect and won't be in this life but have a go at it anyhow.

12. **BE HUMBLE** — Yes, you are great at something. Just don't tell anybody. Let others lift you up.

13. **BE KIND** — Smile wherever you go. It is becoming so rare that it freaks people out (in a good way).

14. **BE GRATEFUL** — Ingratitude is relationship poison. Everyone has worth and something to contribute once you can see past their faults. Try seeing your faults first and work to correct them. Do this before it is too late. We often don't appreciate what we have until it is gone.

15. **BE FORGIVING** — Stop holding grudges. You are just killing yourself—literally. Have the strength to not be easily offended and you will have less forgiving to do.

16. **BE AN EXAMPLE** — When your friends and family see you pulling back from the rat race, some will try talking you out of it — probably because they do not yet have the strength you're showing. You know what is best. Do it. Eventually, a few others might try doing it too.

17. **BE ENDURING** — Divorce rates and for sale signs show us that we chase things we want, get tired of them, and move on to the next "shiny" thing. Be in it for the long haul. Be committed to your commitments.

18. **BE HELPFUL** — Have a heart of service.

19. **BE GENTLE** — The world is full of rage and retaliation. Be the exception.

20. **RADICALLY RELOCATE** — If the gravity your community or situation is too strong, and you cannot escape its orbit, it may be time for a radical relocation. This is a last resort. Thankfully, taking Vitamin "NO" and the rest of your busyness "supplements" makes this maneuver the rarest of options.

STEP 10: RECORD YOUR RESULTS

WRITTEN GOALS AND RESULTS WITH A PLAN OF ACTION KEEP MOTIVATION HIGH AND MAKE SURE HEALTH IS ACHIEVED

In STEP 10 you'll find your daily journal. We made it for 30 days. This section is ultra-important because what gets tracked and measured gets improved upon!

DO NOT BE SURPRISED if the first few days are a little rough. Some detox / withdrawal symptoms are possible. This is normal and expected. Days 3-5 might even be the worst but trust us, it gets easier. Recording the changes helps keep you focused.

It's important to PLAN your meals and TRACK your meals on paper. This will help with proper food types and quantities and to promote food rotation. Remember, if you are trying to lose weight once you hit 50-75g of CARBS for the day...No more! You're done. So, be sure to track your MACROS.

It is also critical to track your TEETER-TOTTER SUPPLEMENTS and your WATER INTAKE to help replenish your nutritional deficiencies.

You need to record your daily RESTERCISE to make sure you keep your heart rate in its proper range (180-AGE). Remember, a high heart rate turns on fight-or-flight and trains the body to stay stressed.

What about SLEEP? Are you getting 8 hours? Are you going to bed by 10 pm? Sleep is as important as any of the other STEPS. So, track that too!

Also, record how you're FEELING THAT DAY. When you listened to your body what did it say? Did a certain food cause bloating/gurgling/gas? Write that down. Did a supplement make you tired or wired? Make a note of that. How was your brain working that day? How was your overall energy? Did the scale drop? Track it.

Another critical question to ask is, "How is my mental health?" Did the events of the day get the best of me? Did you sit for 10-15 minutes and practice being CALM & QUIET? Put it on paper.

Finally, how well are you sticking to the GLUCOSE-GUIDED EATING PLAN? Are certain foods spiking your glucose? Put it on the TIMELINE and find out.

Now, do we think 30 days is all you need to hit your ultimate health goal? Not Likely. This is not a quick fix. It's a lifestyle overhaul so you can experience vitality and longevity.

The good news is enough progress will be made in the first 30 days that motivation will go up. Health and balance will no longer just be goals, they will become your standard. Keep going!

Soon the *50 FIX Plan* will help you overcome adrenaline dominance. The habits and routines of the 10 STEPS will a create "new normal." Adrenaline dominance will no longer have claim to that title.

You have won!

DAY 1:

An object at rest will tend to stay at rest unless it decides to get out of bed.

WATER	SUPPLEMENTS	SNACK	EXERCISE
I DRANK AT LEAST 64 OUNCES OF WATER?	I TOOK ALL OF MY SUPPLEMENTS?	I HAD A PROTEIN SNACK TODAY?	I COMPLETED MY RESTERCISE?
YES ☐ NO ☐	YES ☐ NO ☐	YES ☐ NO ☐	YES ☐ NO ☐

SUN	STRESS	CALM	SLEEP
I GOT 30 MINUTES OF SUN EXPOSURE TOAY?	I MANAGED MY STRESS WELL TODAY?	I TOOK TIME TO BE QUIET AND CALM?	I WILL GET MY 8 HOURS OF SLEEP TONIGHT?
YES ☐ NO ☐	YES ☐ NO ☐	YES ☐ NO ☐	YES ☐ NO ☐

GLUCOSE TIMELINE (record your levels before meals, and optionally at 30 minutes and 2 hours after meals):

6AM 7AM 8AM 9AM 10AM 11AM NOON 1PM 2PM 3PM 4PM 5PM 6PM 7PM 8PM 9PM 10PM 11PM

BREAKFAST:

_____

LUNCH:

_____

DINNER:

_____

NOTES (OVERALL HOW DID I FEEL TODAY?):

_____

_____

_____

DAY 2:

Doubt kills more dreams than failure ever will.

WATER	SUPPLEMENTS	SNACK	EXERCISE
I DRANK AT LEAST 64 OUNCES OF WATER? YES ☐ NO ☐	I TOOK ALL OF MY SUPPLEMENTS? YES ☐ NO ☐	I HAD A PROTEIN SNACK TODAY? YES ☐ NO ☐	I COMPLETED MY RESTERCISE? YES ☐ NO ☐

SUN	STRESS	CALM	SLEEP
I GOT 30 MINUTES OF SUN EXPOSURE TOAY? YES ☐ NO ☐	I MANAGED MY STRESS WELL TODAY? YES ☐ NO ☐	I TOOK TIME TO BE QUIET AND CALM? YES ☐ NO ☐	I WILL GET MY 8 HOURS OF SLEEP TONIGHT? YES ☐ NO ☐

GLUCOSE TIMELINE (record your levels before meals, and optionally at 30 minutes and 2 hours after meals):

6AM 7AM 8AM 9AM 10AM 11AM NOON 1PM 2PM 3PM 4PM 5PM 6PM 7PM 8PM 9PM 10PM 11PM

BREAKFAST:

_____

LUNCH:

_____

DINNER:

_____

NOTES (OVERALL HOW DID I FEEL TODAY?):

_____

_____

_____

DAY 3:

When you change your mindset, you can change your whole world.

WATER	SUPPLEMENTS	SNACK	EXERCISE
I DRANK AT LEAST 64 OUNCES OF WATER?	I TOOK ALL OF MY SUPPLEMENTS?	I HAD A PROTEIN SNACK TODAY?	I COMPLETED MY RESTERCISE?
YES ☐ NO ☐	YES ☐ NO ☐	YES ☐ NO ☐	YES ☐ NO ☐

SUN	STRESS	CALM	SLEEP
I GOT 30 MINUTES OF SUN EXPOSURE TOAY?	I MANAGED MY STRESS WELL TODAY?	I TOOK TIME TO BE QUIET AND CALM?	I WILL GET MY 8 HOURS OF SLEEP TONIGHT?
YES ☐ NO ☐	YES ☐ NO ☐	YES ☐ NO ☐	YES ☐ NO ☐

GLUCOSE TIMELINE (record your levels before meals, and optionally at 30 minutes and 2 hours after meals):

6AM 7AM 8AM 9AM 10AM 11AM NOON 1PM 2PM 3PM 4PM 5PM 6PM 7PM 8PM 9PM 10PM 11PM

BREAKFAST:

_____

LUNCH:

_____

DINNER:

_____

NOTES (OVERALL HOW DID I FEEL TODAY?):

_____

_____

_____

DAY 4:

Life does not get better with random chance; life gets better with intentional change.

WATER	SUPPLEMENTS	SNACK	EXERCISE
I DRANK AT LEAST 64 OUNCES OF WATER?	I TOOK ALL OF MY SUPPLEMENTS?	I HAD A PROTEIN SNACK TODAY?	I COMPLETED MY RESTERCISE?
YES ☐ NO ☐	YES ☐ NO ☐	YES ☐ NO ☐	YES ☐ NO ☐

SUN	STRESS	CALM	SLEEP
I GOT 30 MINUTES OF SUN EXPOSURE TOAY?	I MANAGED MY STRESS WELL TODAY?	I TOOK TIME TO BE QUIET AND CALM?	I WILL GET MY 8 HOURS OF SLEEP TONIGHT?
YES ☐ NO ☐	YES ☐ NO ☐	YES ☐ NO ☐	YES ☐ NO ☐

GLUCOSE TIMELINE (record your levels before meals, and optionally at 30 minutes and 2 hours after meals):

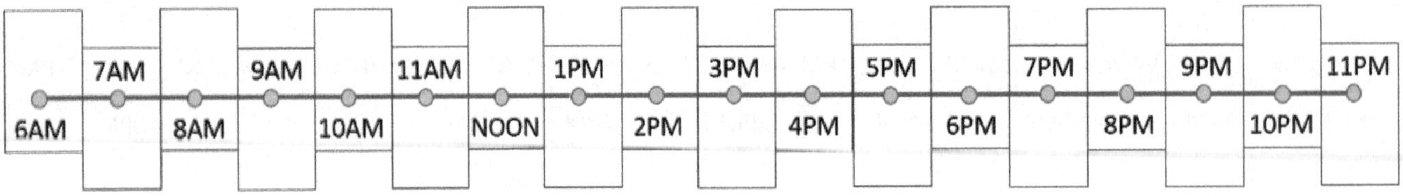

6AM 7AM 8AM 9AM 10AM 11AM NOON 1PM 2PM 3PM 4PM 5PM 6PM 7PM 8PM 9PM 10PM 11PM

BREAKFAST:

_____

LUNCH:

_____

DINNER:

_____

NOTES (OVERALL HOW DID I FEEL TODAY?):

_____

_____

_____

DAY 5:

Focus on what you want, but always be grateful for what you have.

WATER	SUPPLEMENTS	SNACK	EXERCISE
I DRANK AT LEAST 64 OUNCES OF WATER?	I TOOK ALL OF MY SUPPLEMENTS?	I HAD A PROTEIN SNACK TODAY?	I COMPLETED MY RESTERCISE?
YES ☐ NO ☐	YES ☐ NO ☐	YES ☐ NO ☐	YES ☐ NO ☐

SUN	STRESS	CALM	SLEEP
I GOT 30 MINUTES OF SUN EXPOSURE TOAY?	I MANAGED MY STRESS WELL TODAY?	I TOOK TIME TO BE QUIET AND CALM?	I WILL GET MY 8 HOURS OF SLEEP TONIGHT?
YES ☐ NO ☐	YES ☐ NO ☐	YES ☐ NO ☐	YES ☐ NO ☐

GLUCOSE TIMELINE (record your levels before meals, and optionally at 30 minutes and 2 hours after meals):

6AM · 7AM · 8AM · 9AM · 10AM · 11AM · NOON · 1PM · 2PM · 3PM · 4PM · 5PM · 6PM · 7PM · 8PM · 9PM · 10PM · 11PM

BREAKFAST:

_____

LUNCH:

_____

DINNER:

_____

NOTES (OVERALL HOW DID I FEEL TODAY?):

_____

_____

_____

DAY 6:

Motivation determines what you do; attitude determines how well you do it.

WATER	SUPPLEMENTS	SNACK	EXERCISE
I DRANK AT LEAST 64 OUNCES OF WATER?	I TOOK ALL OF MY SUPPLEMENTS?	I HAD A PROTEIN SNACK TODAY?	I COMPLETED MY RESTERCISE?
YES ☐ NO ☐	YES ☐ NO ☐	YES ☐ NO ☐	YES ☐ NO ☐

SUN	STRESS	CALM	SLEEP
I GOT 30 MINUTES OF SUN EXPOSURE TOAY?	I MANAGED MY STRESS WELL TODAY?	I TOOK TIME TO BE QUIET AND CALM?	I WILL GET MY 8 HOURS OF SLEEP TONIGHT?
YES ☐ NO ☐	YES ☐ NO ☐	YES ☐ NO ☐	YES ☐ NO ☐

GLUCOSE TIMELINE (record your levels before meals, and optionally at 30 minutes and 2 hours after meals):

6AM 7AM 8AM 9AM 10AM 11AM NOON 1PM 2PM 3PM 4PM 5PM 6PM 7PM 8PM 9PM 10PM 11PM

BREAKFAST:

_____

LUNCH:

_____

DINNER:

_____

NOTES (OVERALL HOW DID I FEEL TODAY?):

_____

_____

_____

DAY 7:

Sometime later, becomes never; Do it now.

WATER	SUPPLEMENTS	SNACK	EXERCISE
I DRANK AT LEAST 64 OUNCES OF WATER?	I TOOK ALL OF MY SUPPLEMENTS?	I HAD A PROTEIN SNACK TODAY?	I COMPLETED MY RESTERCISE?
YES ☐ NO ☐	YES ☐ NO ☐	YES ☐ NO ☐	YES ☐ NO ☐

SUN	STRESS	CALM	SLEEP
I GOT 30 MINUTES OF SUN EXPOSURE TOAY?	I MANAGED MY STRESS WELL TODAY?	I TOOK TIME TO BE QUIET AND CALM?	I WILL GET MY 8 HOURS OF SLEEP TONIGHT?
YES ☐ NO ☐	YES ☐ NO ☐	YES ☐ NO ☐	YES ☐ NO ☐

GLUCOSE TIMELINE (record your levels before meals, and optionally at 30 minutes and 2 hours after meals):

6AM 7AM 8AM 9AM 10AM 11AM NOON 1PM 2PM 3PM 4PM 5PM 6PM 7PM 8PM 9PM 10PM 11PM

BREAKFAST:

_____

LUNCH:

_____

DINNER:

_____

NOTES (OVERALL HOW DID I FEEL TODAY?):

_____

_____

_____

DAY 8:

The best way to predict the future is to create it.

WATER	SUPPLEMENTS	SNACK	EXERCISE
I DRANK AT LEAST 64 OUNCES OF WATER?	I TOOK ALL OF MY SUPPLEMENTS?	I HAD A PROTEIN SNACK TODAY?	I COMPLETED MY RESTERCISE?
YES ☐ NO ☐	YES ☐ NO ☐	YES ☐ NO ☐	YES ☐ NO ☐

SUN	STRESS	CALM	SLEEP
I GOT 30 MINUTES OF SUN EXPOSURE TOAY?	I MANAGED MY STRESS WELL TODAY?	I TOOK TIME TO BE QUIET AND CALM?	I WILL GET MY 8 HOURS OF SLEEP TONIGHT?
YES ☐ NO ☐	YES ☐ NO ☐	YES ☐ NO ☐	YES ☐ NO ☐

GLUCOSE TIMELINE (record your levels before meals, and optionally at 30 minutes and 2 hours after meals):

6AM 7AM 8AM 9AM 10AM 11AM NOON 1PM 2PM 3PM 4PM 5PM 6PM 7PM 8PM 9PM 10PM 11PM

BREAKFAST:

_____

LUNCH:

_____

DINNER:

_____

NOTES (OVERALL HOW DID I FEEL TODAY?):

_____

_____

_____

DAY 9:

Obstacles are what you see when your eyes are not on the goal.

WATER	SUPPLEMENTS	SNACK	EXERCISE
I DRANK AT LEAST 64 OUNCES OF WATER?	I TOOK ALL OF MY SUPPLEMENTS?	I HAD A PROTEIN SNACK TODAY?	I COMPLETED MY RESTERCISE?
YES ☐ NO ☐	YES ☐ NO ☐	YES ☐ NO ☐	YES ☐ NO ☐

SUN	STRESS	CALM	SLEEP
I GOT 30 MINUTES OF SUN EXPOSURE TOAY?	I MANAGED MY STRESS WELL TODAY?	I TOOK TIME TO BE QUIET AND CALM?	I WILL GET MY 8 HOURS OF SLEEP TONIGHT?
YES ☐ NO ☐	YES ☐ NO ☐	YES ☐ NO ☐	YES ☐ NO ☐

GLUCOSE TIMELINE (record your levels before meals, and optionally at 30 minutes and 2 hours after meals):

6AM 7AM 8AM 9AM 10AM 11AM NOON 1PM 2PM 3PM 4PM 5PM 6PM 7PM 8PM 9PM 10PM 11PM

BREAKFAST:

_____

LUNCH:

_____

DINNER:

_____

NOTES (OVERALL HOW DID I FEEL TODAY?):

_____
_____
_____

DAY 10:

Only you can change your life; no one else can do it for you.

WATER	SUPPLEMENTS	SNACK	EXERCISE
I DRANK AT LEAST 64 OUNCES OF WATER?	I TOOK ALL OF MY SUPPLEMENTS?	I HAD A PROTEIN SNACK TODAY?	I COMPLETED MY RESTERCISE?
YES ☐ NO ☐	YES ☐ NO ☐	YES ☐ NO ☐	YES ☐ NO ☐

SUN	STRESS	CALM	SLEEP
I GOT 30 MINUTES OF SUN EXPOSURE TOAY?	I MANAGED MY STRESS WELL TODAY?	I TOOK TIME TO BE QUIET AND CALM?	I WILL GET MY 8 HOURS OF SLEEP TONIGHT?
YES ☐ NO ☐	YES ☐ NO ☐	YES ☐ NO ☐	YES ☐ NO ☐

GLUCOSE TIMELINE (record your levels before meals, and optionally at 30 minutes and 2 hours after meals):

6AM 7AM 8AM 9AM 10AM 11AM NOON 1PM 2PM 3PM 4PM 5PM 6PM 7PM 8PM 9PM 10PM 11PM

BREAKFAST:

_____

LUNCH:

_____

DINNER:

_____

NOTES (OVERALL HOW DID I FEEL TODAY?):

_____

_____

_____

DAY 11:

If you change the way you look at things, the things you look at change.

WATER	SUPPLEMENTS	SNACK	EXERCISE
I DRANK AT LEAST 64 OUNCES OF WATER?	I TOOK ALL OF MY SUPPLEMENTS?	I HAD A PROTEIN SNACK TODAY?	I COMPLETED MY RESTERCISE?
YES ☐ NO ☐	YES ☐ NO ☐	YES ☐ NO ☐	YES ☐ NO ☐

SUN	STRESS	CALM	SLEEP
I GOT 30 MINUTES OF SUN EXPOSURE TOAY?	I MANAGED MY STRESS WELL TODAY?	I TOOK TIME TO BE QUIET AND CALM?	I WILL GET MY 8 HOURS OF SLEEP TONIGHT?
YES ☐ NO ☐	YES ☐ NO ☐	YES ☐ NO ☐	YES ☐ NO ☐

GLUCOSE TIMELINE (record your levels before meals, and optionally at 30 minutes and 2 hours after meals):

6AM 7AM 8AM 9AM 10AM 11AM NOON 1PM 2PM 3PM 4PM 5PM 6PM 7PM 8PM 9PM 10PM 11PM

BREAKFAST:

_____

LUNCH:

_____

DINNER:

_____

NOTES (OVERALL HOW DID I FEEL TODAY?):

_____

_____

_____

DAY 12:

Courage doesn't mean you don't get afraid; courage means you don't let fear stop you.

WATER	SUPPLEMENTS	SNACK	EXERCISE
I DRANK AT LEAST 64 OUNCES OF WATER?	I TOOK ALL OF MY SUPPLEMENTS?	I HAD A PROTEIN SNACK TODAY?	I COMPLETED MY RESTERCISE?
YES ☐ NO ☐	YES ☐ NO ☐	YES ☐ NO ☐	YES ☐ NO ☐

SUN	STRESS	CALM	SLEEP
I GOT 30 MINUTES OF SUN EXPOSURE TOAY?	I MANAGED MY STRESS WELL TODAY?	I TOOK TIME TO BE QUIET AND CALM?	I WILL GET MY 8 HOURS OF SLEEP TONIGHT?
YES ☐ NO ☐	YES ☐ NO ☐	YES ☐ NO ☐	YES ☐ NO ☐

GLUCOSE TIMELINE (record your levels before meals, and optionally at 30 minutes and 2 hours after meals):

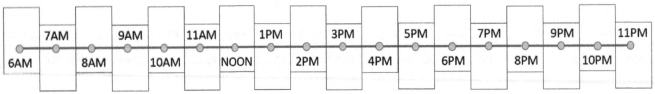

BREAKFAST:

_____

LUNCH:

_____

DINNER:

_____

NOTES (OVERALL HOW DID I FEEL TODAY?):

_____

_____

_____

DAY 13:

Strength doesn't come by what you can do; it comes by overcoming what you thought you couldn't.

WATER	SUPPLEMENTS	SNACK	EXERCISE
I DRANK AT LEAST 64 OUNCES OF WATER?	I TOOK ALL OF MY SUPPLEMENTS?	I HAD A PROTEIN SNACK TODAY?	I COMPLETED MY RESTERCISE?
YES ☐ NO ☐	YES ☐ NO ☐	YES ☐ NO ☐	YES ☐ NO ☐

SUN	STRESS	CALM	SLEEP
I GOT 30 MINUTES OF SUN EXPOSURE TOAY?	I MANAGED MY STRESS WELL TODAY?	I TOOK TIME TO BE QUIET AND CALM?	I WILL GET MY 8 HOURS OF SLEEP TONIGHT?
YES ☐ NO ☐	YES ☐ NO ☐	YES ☐ NO ☐	YES ☐ NO ☐

GLUCOSE TIMELINE (record your levels before meals, and optionally at 30 minutes and 2 hours after meals):

6AM 7AM 8AM 9AM 10AM 11AM NOON 1PM 2PM 3PM 4PM 5PM 6PM 7PM 8PM 9PM 10PM 11PM

BREAKFAST:

_____

LUNCH:

_____

DINNER:

_____

NOTES (OVERALL HOW DID I FEEL TODAY?):

_____
_____
_____

DAY 14:

Start strong, stay strong, finish strong, by remembering why you started in the first place.

WATER	SUPPLEMENTS	SNACK	EXERCISE
I DRANK AT LEAST 64 OUNCES OF WATER?	I TOOK ALL OF MY SUPPLEMENTS?	I HAD A PROTEIN SNACK TODAY?	I COMPLETED MY RESTERCISE?
YES ☐ NO ☐	YES ☐ NO ☐	YES ☐ NO ☐	YES ☐ NO ☐

SUN	STRESS	CALM	SLEEP
I GOT 30 MINUTES OF SUN EXPOSURE TOAY?	I MANAGED MY STRESS WELL TODAY?	I TOOK TIME TO BE QUIET AND CALM?	I WILL GET MY 8 HOURS OF SLEEP TONIGHT?
YES ☐ NO ☐	YES ☐ NO ☐	YES ☐ NO ☐	YES ☐ NO ☐

GLUCOSE TIMELINE (record your levels before meals, and optionally at 30 minutes and 2 hours after meals):

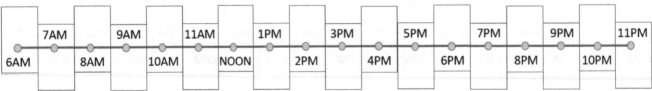

6AM 7AM 8AM 9AM 10AM 11AM NOON 1PM 2PM 3PM 4PM 5PM 6PM 7PM 8PM 9PM 10PM 11PM

BREAKFAST:

_____

LUNCH:

_____

DINNER:

_____

NOTES (OVERALL HOW DID I FEEL TODAY?):

_____

_____

_____

DAY 15:

Believe you can and you're halfway there.

WATER	SUPPLEMENTS	SNACK	EXERCISE
I DRANK AT LEAST 64 OUNCES OF WATER?	I TOOK ALL OF MY SUPPLEMENTS?	I HAD A PROTEIN SNACK TODAY?	I COMPLETED MY RESTERCISE?
YES ☐ NO ☐	YES ☐ NO ☐	YES ☐ NO ☐	YES ☐ NO ☐

SUN	STRESS	CALM	SLEEP
I GOT 30 MINUTES OF SUN EXPOSURE TOAY?	I MANAGED MY STRESS WELL TODAY?	I TOOK TIME TO BE QUIET AND CALM?	I WILL GET MY 8 HOURS OF SLEEP TONIGHT?
YES ☐ NO ☐	YES ☐ NO ☐	YES ☐ NO ☐	YES ☐ NO ☐

GLUCOSE TIMELINE (record your levels before meals, and optionally at 30 minutes and 2 hours after meals):

6AM 7AM 8AM 9AM 10AM 11AM NOON 1PM 2PM 3PM 4PM 5PM 6PM 7PM 8PM 9PM 10PM 11PM

BREAKFAST:

_____

LUNCH:

_____

DINNER:

_____

NOTES (OVERALL HOW DID I FEEL TODAY?):

_____

_____

_____

DAY 16:

Do today what your future self will thank you for.

WATER	SUPPLEMENTS	SNACK	EXERCISE
I DRANK AT LEAST 64 OUNCES OF WATER?	I TOOK ALL OF MY SUPPLEMENTS?	I HAD A PROTEIN SNACK TODAY?	I COMPLETED MY RESTERCISE?
YES ☐ NO ☐	YES ☐ NO ☐	YES ☐ NO ☐	YES ☐ NO ☐

SUN	STRESS	CALM	SLEEP
I GOT 30 MINUTES OF SUN EXPOSURE TOAY?	I MANAGED MY STRESS WELL TODAY?	I TOOK TIME TO BE QUIET AND CALM?	I WILL GET MY 8 HOURS OF SLEEP TONIGHT?
YES ☐ NO ☐	YES ☐ NO ☐	YES ☐ NO ☐	YES ☐ NO ☐

GLUCOSE TIMELINE (record your levels before meals, and optionally at 30 minutes and 2 hours after meals):

6AM — 7AM — 8AM — 9AM — 10AM — 11AM — NOON — 1PM — 2PM — 3PM — 4PM — 5PM — 6PM — 7PM — 8PM — 9PM — 10PM — 11PM

BREAKFAST:

_____

LUNCH:

_____

DINNER:

_____

NOTES (OVERALL HOW DID I FEEL TODAY?):

_____

_____

_____

DAY 17:

When you feel like quitting, think about why you started.

WATER	SUPPLEMENTS	SNACK	EXERCISE
I DRANK AT LEAST 64 OUNCES OF WATER?	I TOOK ALL OF MY SUPPLEMENTS?	I HAD A PROTEIN SNACK TODAY?	I COMPLETED MY RESTERCISE?
YES ☐ NO ☐	YES ☐ NO ☐	YES ☐ NO ☐	YES ☐ NO ☐

SUN	STRESS	CALM	SLEEP
I GOT 30 MINUTES OF SUN EXPOSURE TOAY?	I MANAGED MY STRESS WELL TODAY?	I TOOK TIME TO BE QUIET AND CALM?	I WILL GET MY 8 HOURS OF SLEEP TONIGHT?
YES ☐ NO ☐	YES ☐ NO ☐	YES ☐ NO ☐	YES ☐ NO ☐

GLUCOSE TIMELINE (record your levels before meals, and optionally at 30 minutes and 2 hours after meals):

6AM 7AM 8AM 9AM 10AM 11AM NOON 1PM 2PM 3PM 4PM 5PM 6PM 7PM 8PM 9PM 10PM 11PM

BREAKFAST:

_____

LUNCH:

_____

DINNER:

_____

NOTES (OVERALL HOW DID I FEEL TODAY?):

_____
_____
_____

DAY 18:

Keep your face toward the sunshine and the shadows will always be behind you.

WATER	SUPPLEMENTS	SNACK	EXERCISE
I DRANK AT LEAST 64 OUNCES OF WATER?	I TOOK ALL OF MY SUPPLEMENTS?	I HAD A PROTEIN SNACK TODAY?	I COMPLETED MY RESTERCISE?
YES ☐ NO ☐	YES ☐ NO ☐	YES ☐ NO ☐	YES ☐ NO ☐

SUN	STRESS	CALM	SLEEP
I GOT 30 MINUTES OF SUN EXPOSURE TOAY?	I MANAGED MY STRESS WELL TODAY?	I TOOK TIME TO BE QUIET AND CALM?	I WILL GET MY 8 HOURS OF SLEEP TONIGHT?
YES ☐ NO ☐	YES ☐ NO ☐	YES ☐ NO ☐	YES ☐ NO ☐

GLUCOSE TIMELINE (record your levels before meals, and optionally at 30 minutes and 2 hours after meals):

6AM 7AM 8AM 9AM 10AM 11AM NOON 1PM 2PM 3PM 4PM 5PM 6PM 7PM 8PM 9PM 10PM 11PM

BREAKFAST:

_____

LUNCH:

_____

DINNER:

_____

NOTES (OVERALL HOW DID I FEEL TODAY?):

_____
_____
_____

DAY 19:

Focusing on results does not guarantee change; focusing on change guarantees results.

WATER	SUPPLEMENTS	SNACK	EXERCISE
I DRANK AT LEAST 64 OUNCES OF WATER?	I TOOK ALL OF MY SUPPLEMENTS?	I HAD A PROTEIN SNACK TODAY?	I COMPLETED MY RESTERCISE?
YES ☐ NO ☐	YES ☐ NO ☐	YES ☐ NO ☐	YES ☐ NO ☐

SUN	STRESS	CALM	SLEEP
I GOT 30 MINUTES OF SUN EXPOSURE TOAY?	I MANAGED MY STRESS WELL TODAY?	I TOOK TIME TO BE QUIET AND CALM?	I WILL GET MY 8 HOURS OF SLEEP TONIGHT?
YES ☐ NO ☐	YES ☐ NO ☐	YES ☐ NO ☐	YES ☐ NO ☐

GLUCOSE TIMELINE (record your levels before meals, and optionally at 30 minutes and 2 hours after meals):

6AM 7AM 8AM 9AM 10AM 11AM NOON 1PM 2PM 3PM 4PM 5PM 6PM 7PM 8PM 9PM 10PM 11PM

BREAKFAST:

_____

LUNCH:

_____

DINNER:

_____

NOTES (OVERALL HOW DID I FEEL TODAY?):

_____

_____

_____

DAY 20:

If the little things are done daily, the hard things will get done.

WATER	SUPPLEMENTS	SNACK	EXERCISE
I DRANK AT LEAST 64 OUNCES OF WATER?	I TOOK ALL OF MY SUPPLEMENTS?	I HAD A PROTEIN SNACK TODAY?	I COMPLETED MY RESTERCISE?
YES ☐ NO ☐	YES ☐ NO ☐	YES ☐ NO ☐	YES ☐ NO ☐

SUN	STRESS	CALM	SLEEP
I GOT 30 MINUTES OF SUN EXPOSURE TOAY?	I MANAGED MY STRESS WELL TODAY?	I TOOK TIME TO BE QUIET AND CALM?	I WILL GET MY 8 HOURS OF SLEEP TONIGHT?
YES ☐ NO ☐	YES ☐ NO ☐	YES ☐ NO ☐	YES ☐ NO ☐

GLUCOSE TIMELINE (record your levels before meals, and optionally at 30 minutes and 2 hours after meals):

6AM 7AM 8AM 9AM 10AM 11AM NOON 1PM 2PM 3PM 4PM 5PM 6PM 7PM 8PM 9PM 10PM 11PM

BREAKFAST:

_____

LUNCH:

_____

DINNER:

_____

NOTES (OVERALL HOW DID I FEEL TODAY?):

_____

_____

_____

DAY 21:

Every day may not be good, but there is something good in every day.

WATER	SUPPLEMENTS	SNACK	EXERCISE
I DRANK AT LEAST 64 OUNCES OF WATER?	I TOOK ALL OF MY SUPPLEMENTS?	I HAD A PROTEIN SNACK TODAY?	I COMPLETED MY RESTERCISE?
YES ☐ NO ☐	YES ☐ NO ☐	YES ☐ NO ☐	YES ☐ NO ☐

SUN	STRESS	CALM	SLEEP
I GOT 30 MINUTES OF SUN EXPOSURE TOAY?	I MANAGED MY STRESS WELL TODAY?	I TOOK TIME TO BE QUIET AND CALM?	I WILL GET MY 8 HOURS OF SLEEP TONIGHT?
YES ☐ NO ☐	YES ☐ NO ☐	YES ☐ NO ☐	YES ☐ NO ☐

GLUCOSE TIMELINE (record your levels before meals, and optionally at 30 minutes and 2 hours after meals):

6AM	7AM	8AM	9AM	10AM	11AM	NOON	1PM	2PM	3PM	4PM	5PM	6PM	7PM	8PM	9PM	10PM	11PM

BREAKFAST:

_____

LUNCH:

_____

DINNER:

_____

NOTES (OVERALL HOW DID I FEEL TODAY?):

_____

_____

_____

DAY 22:

If it doesn't challenge you, it doesn't change you.

WATER	SUPPLEMENTS	SNACK	EXERCISE
I DRANK AT LEAST 64 OUNCES OF WATER?	I TOOK ALL OF MY SUPPLEMENTS?	I HAD A PROTEIN SNACK TODAY?	I COMPLETED MY RESTERCISE?
YES ☐ NO ☐	YES ☐ NO ☐	YES ☐ NO ☐	YES ☐ NO ☐

SUN	STRESS	CALM	SLEEP
I GOT 30 MINUTES OF SUN EXPOSURE TOAY?	I MANAGED MY STRESS WELL TODAY?	I TOOK TIME TO BE QUIET AND CALM?	I WILL GET MY 8 HOURS OF SLEEP TONIGHT?
YES ☐ NO ☐	YES ☐ NO ☐	YES ☐ NO ☐	YES ☐ NO ☐

GLUCOSE TIMELINE (record your levels before meals, and optionally at 30 minutes and 2 hours after meals):

6AM 7AM 8AM 9AM 10AM 11AM NOON 1PM 2PM 3PM 4PM 5PM 6PM 7PM 8PM 9PM 10PM 11PM

BREAKFAST:

_____

LUNCH:

_____

DINNER:

_____

NOTES (OVERALL HOW DID I FEEL TODAY?):

_____
_____
_____

DAY 23:

Climb mountains not so the world can see you, but so you can see a new world.

WATER I DRANK AT LEAST 64 OUNCES OF WATER? YES ☐ NO ☐	**SUPPLEMENTS** I TOOK ALL OF MY SUPPLEMENTS? YES ☐ NO ☐	**SNACK** I HAD A PROTEIN SNACK TODAY? YES ☐ NO ☐	**EXERCISE** I COMPLETED MY RESTERCISE? YES ☐ NO ☐
SUN I GOT 30 MINUTES OF SUN EXPOSURE TOAY? YES ☐ NO ☐	**STRESS** I MANAGED MY STRESS WELL TODAY? YES ☐ NO ☐	**CALM** I TOOK TIME TO BE QUIET AND CALM? YES ☐ NO ☐	**SLEEP** I WILL GET MY 8 HOURS OF SLEEP TONIGHT? YES ☐ NO ☐

GLUCOSE TIMELINE (record your levels before meals, and optionally at 30 minutes and 2 hours after meals):

6AM 7AM 8AM 9AM 10AM 11AM NOON 1PM 2PM 3PM 4PM 5PM 6PM 7PM 8PM 9PM 10PM 11PM

BREAKFAST:

_____

LUNCH:

_____

DINNER:

_____

NOTES (OVERALL HOW DID I FEEL TODAY?):

_____

_____

_____

DAY 24:

Motivation is what gets you started; habits are what keep you going.

WATER	SUPPLEMENTS	SNACK	EXERCISE
I DRANK AT LEAST 64 OUNCES OF WATER?	I TOOK ALL OF MY SUPPLEMENTS?	I HAD A PROTEIN SNACK TODAY?	I COMPLETED MY RESTERCISE?
YES ☐ NO ☐	YES ☐ NO ☐	YES ☐ NO ☐	YES ☐ NO ☐

SUN	STRESS	CALM	SLEEP
I GOT 30 MINUTES OF SUN EXPOSURE TOAY?	I MANAGED MY STRESS WELL TODAY?	I TOOK TIME TO BE QUIET AND CALM?	I WILL GET MY 8 HOURS OF SLEEP TONIGHT?
YES ☐ NO ☐	YES ☐ NO ☐	YES ☐ NO ☐	YES ☐ NO ☐

GLUCOSE TIMELINE (record your levels before meals, and optionally at 30 minutes and 2 hours after meals):

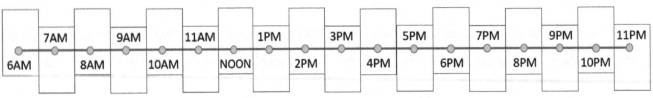

BREAKFAST:

_____

LUNCH:

_____

DINNER:

_____

NOTES (OVERALL HOW DID I FEEL TODAY?):

_____

_____

_____

DAY 25:

You only live once; if done right, once is enough.

WATER	SUPPLEMENTS	SNACK	EXERCISE
I DRANK AT LEAST 64 OUNCES OF WATER?	I TOOK ALL OF MY SUPPLEMENTS?	I HAD A PROTEIN SNACK TODAY?	I COMPLETED MY RESTERCISE?
YES ☐ NO ☐	YES ☐ NO ☐	YES ☐ NO ☐	YES ☐ NO ☐

SUN	STRESS	CALM	SLEEP
I GOT 30 MINUTES OF SUN EXPOSURE TOAY?	I MANAGED MY STRESS WELL TODAY?	I TOOK TIME TO BE QUIET AND CALM?	I WILL GET MY 8 HOURS OF SLEEP TONIGHT?
YES ☐ NO ☐	YES ☐ NO ☐	YES ☐ NO ☐	YES ☐ NO ☐

GLUCOSE TIMELINE (record your levels before meals, and optionally at 30 minutes and 2 hours after meals):

6AM 7AM 8AM 9AM 10AM 11AM NOON 1PM 2PM 3PM 4PM 5PM 6PM 7PM 8PM 9PM 10PM 11PM

BREAKFAST:

_____

LUNCH:

_____

DINNER:

_____

NOTES (OVERALL HOW DID I FEEL TODAY?):

_____

_____

_____

DAY 26:

I CAN is far superior to IQ.

WATER	SUPPLEMENTS	SNACK	EXERCISE
I DRANK AT LEAST 64 OUNCES OF WATER?	I TOOK ALL OF MY SUPPLEMENTS?	I HAD A PROTEIN SNACK TODAY?	I COMPLETED MY RESTERCISE?
YES ☐ NO ☐	YES ☐ NO ☐	YES ☐ NO ☐	YES ☐ NO ☐

SUN	STRESS	CALM	SLEEP
I GOT 30 MINUTES OF SUN EXPOSURE TOAY?	I MANAGED MY STRESS WELL TODAY?	I TOOK TIME TO BE QUIET AND CALM?	I WILL GET MY 8 HOURS OF SLEEP TONIGHT?
YES ☐ NO ☐	YES ☐ NO ☐	YES ☐ NO ☐	YES ☐ NO ☐

GLUCOSE TIMELINE (record your levels before meals, and optionally at 30 minutes and 2 hours after meals):

6AM 7AM 8AM 9AM 10AM 11AM NOON 1PM 2PM 3PM 4PM 5PM 6PM 7PM 8PM 9PM 10PM 11PM

BREAKFAST:

_____

LUNCH:

_____

DINNER:

_____

NOTES (OVERALL HOW DID I FEEL TODAY?):

_____

_____

_____

DAY 27:

Fear of the mountain makes it grow; climbing the mountain makes you grow.

WATER	SUPPLEMENTS	SNACK	EXERCISE
I DRANK AT LEAST 64 OUNCES OF WATER?	I TOOK ALL OF MY SUPPLEMENTS?	I HAD A PROTEIN SNACK TODAY?	I COMPLETED MY RESTERCISE?
YES ☐ NO ☐	YES ☐ NO ☐	YES ☐ NO ☐	YES ☐ NO ☐

SUN	STRESS	CALM	SLEEP
I GOT 30 MINUTES OF SUN EXPOSURE TOAY?	I MANAGED MY STRESS WELL TODAY?	I TOOK TIME TO BE QUIET AND CALM?	I WILL GET MY 8 HOURS OF SLEEP TONIGHT?
YES ☐ NO ☐	YES ☐ NO ☐	YES ☐ NO ☐	YES ☐ NO ☐

GLUCOSE TIMELINE (record your levels before meals, and optionally at 30 minutes and 2 hours after meals):

6AM 7AM 8AM 9AM 10AM 11AM NOON 1PM 2PM 3PM 4PM 5PM 6PM 7PM 8PM 9PM 10PM 11PM

BREAKFAST:

_____

LUNCH:

_____

DINNER:

_____

NOTES (OVERALL HOW DID I FEEL TODAY?):

_____
_____
_____

DAY 28:

Don't count the days; make the days count.

WATER	SUPPLEMENTS	SNACK	EXERCISE
I DRANK AT LEAST 64 OUNCES OF WATER?	I TOOK ALL OF MY SUPPLEMENTS?	I HAD A PROTEIN SNACK TODAY?	I COMPLETED MY RESTERCISE?
YES ☐ NO ☐	YES ☐ NO ☐	YES ☐ NO ☐	YES ☐ NO ☐

SUN	STRESS	CALM	SLEEP
I GOT 30 MINUTES OF SUN EXPOSURE TOAY?	I MANAGED MY STRESS WELL TODAY?	I TOOK TIME TO BE QUIET AND CALM?	I WILL GET MY 8 HOURS OF SLEEP TONIGHT?
YES ☐ NO ☐	YES ☐ NO ☐	YES ☐ NO ☐	YES ☐ NO ☐

GLUCOSE TIMELINE (record your levels before meals, and optionally at 30 minutes and 2 hours after meals):

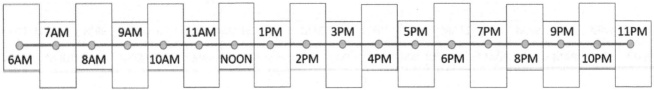

BREAKFAST:

_____

LUNCH:

_____

DINNER:

_____

NOTES (OVERALL HOW DID I FEEL TODAY?):

_____

_____

_____

DAY 29:

Habits from discipline produce the fruit of success; motivation from desperation is the fruit of regrets

WATER	SUPPLEMENTS	SNACK	EXERCISE
I DRANK AT LEAST 64 OUNCES OF WATER?	I TOOK ALL OF MY SUPPLEMENTS?	I HAD A PROTEIN SNACK TODAY?	I COMPLETED MY RESTERCISE?
YES ☐ NO ☐	YES ☐ NO ☐	YES ☐ NO ☐	YES ☐ NO ☐

SUN	STRESS	CALM	SLEEP
I GOT 30 MINUTES OF SUN EXPOSURE TOAY?	I MANAGED MY STRESS WELL TODAY?	I TOOK TIME TO BE QUIET AND CALM?	I WILL GET MY 8 HOURS OF SLEEP TONIGHT?
YES ☐ NO ☐	YES ☐ NO ☐	YES ☐ NO ☐	YES ☐ NO ☐

GLUCOSE TIMELINE (record your levels before meals, and optionally at 30 minutes and 2 hours after meals):

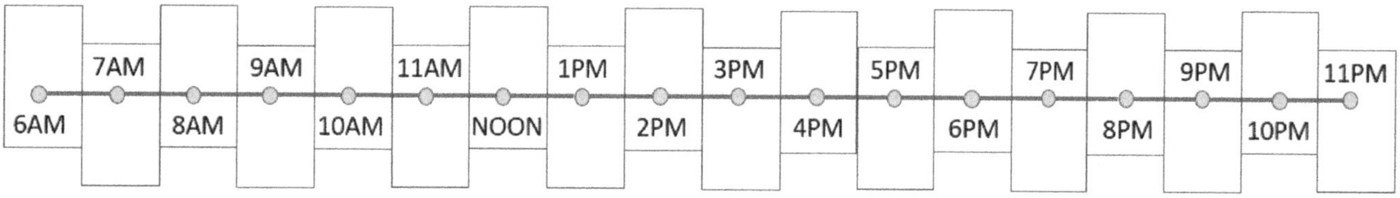

6AM 7AM 8AM 9AM 10AM 11AM NOON 1PM 2PM 3PM 4PM 5PM 6PM 7PM 8PM 9PM 10PM 11PM

BREAKFAST:

_____

LUNCH:

_____

DINNER:

_____

NOTES (OVERALL HOW DID I FEEL TODAY?):

_____

_____

_____

DAY 30:

Healthy is an outfit that looks different on everybody.

WATER	SUPPLEMENTS	SNACK	EXERCISE
I DRANK AT LEAST 64 OUNCES OF WATER?	I TOOK ALL OF MY SUPPLEMENTS?	I HAD A PROTEIN SNACK TODAY?	I COMPLETED MY RESTERCISE?
YES ☐ NO ☐	YES ☐ NO ☐	YES ☐ NO ☐	YES ☐ NO ☐

SUN	STRESS	CALM	SLEEP
I GOT 30 MINUTES OF SUN EXPOSURE TOAY?	I MANAGED MY STRESS WELL TODAY?	I TOOK TIME TO BE QUIET AND CALM?	I WILL GET MY 8 HOURS OF SLEEP TONIGHT?
YES ☐ NO ☐	YES ☐ NO ☐	YES ☐ NO ☐	YES ☐ NO ☐

GLUCOSE TIMELINE (record your levels before meals, and optionally at 30 minutes and 2 hours after meals):

6AM 7AM 8AM 9AM 10AM 11AM NOON 1PM 2PM 3PM 4PM 5PM 6PM 7PM 8PM 9PM 10PM 11PM

BREAKFAST:

_____

LUNCH:

_____

DINNER:

_____

NOTES (OVERALL HOW DID I FEEL TODAY?):

_____
_____
_____

PART 3: THE EFFECTS OF ADRENALINE DOMINACE

You have come a long way. By now you have looked over the entire *50 FIX Plan*. This means you have what you need to balance your CORE4 and make major positive shifts in your health. However, no plan works unless it is followed. To get started and to stay on the *50 FIX Plan* requires daily motivation.

PART 3 is all about education for motivation. On the *50 FIX Plan* you will already be motivated by the data from your labs, your daily glucose testing, and the tracking of your *Restercise* and overall progress. Now, a little immersion here in PART 3 will also help to keep motivation high.

Although no system of the body is exempt from the wrath of adrenaline dominance, below I focus on some details of three body systems—digestive, hormonal, and immune—and just some of their common ailments.

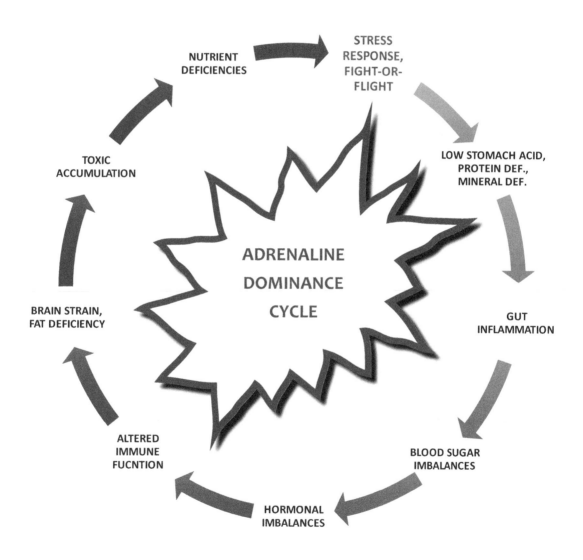

DIGESTIVE TRACT

IT STARTS IN THE MOUTH

Digestive issues and most chronic illnesses start in the mouth. What we eat, drink, and breathe has immediate positive or negative effects on every system of the body. For the internal organs to function their best, detoxify and stay healthy, they require proper nutrients, which must come from the diet. So, when food does more harm than good, not only are the required resources lacking, but the body's nutritional reserves are drained to manage the processing of unhealthy food. In a short period of time these resources come to an end and adrenaline surges begin.

IT STARTS WHEN THEY ARE YOUNG

If a mom has spent her prenatal life suffering from digestive upset, anxiety, acne, and PMS, it is a near guarantee that she has been eating the wrong foods for her body. As a result, her blood became full of excess chemical waste products from her inflamed gut and over-active immune system. These toxins help stoke an adrenaline fire. Now mom can add anxiety to her symptom menu and so can her child. According to many studies, maternal anxiety directly leads to cognitive, behavioral, and emotional problems in the child.[48] Immune compromised mothers are giving birth to immune compromised children.

The digestive issues in the child are nearly immediate. Babies that are overly fussy, have colic or spit up after most meals, babies that do not have several bowel movements a day or have no bowel movements for several days, as well as babies whose stools are loose and green, are all experiencing digestive disruptions. More specifically, they are not efficiently processing mama's milk or bottle formula. These problems are very common. But that does not make them normal. Quite the opposite.

> I have helped hundreds of children with these issues simply by modifying their diets and providing a few supplements. Typically, within one or two visits their symptoms are gone thanks to the correct whole-person approach and the inspiring ability of the body to heal itself.

THE SNOWBALL EFFECT

The toddler who still eats the same gut-irritating and inflaming foods will often throw tantrums, have skin issues, (big rosy cheeks and rashes on their belly or arms) complain of stomach aches, struggle to sleep, and later also experience growing pains or muscle cramps. Since sixty percent of the immune system is in the digestive tract, the child commonly begins having allergies or asthma, catches colds, gets ear infections, and maybe strep throat. Antibiotics are introduced to fight off the infections, which also kill the good bacteria in the gut. Now a gut that was already inflamed from improper foods or that started off compromised, is potentially made much worse. Antibiotic use is associated with the proliferation and virulence of pathogens, leaky gut syndrome, and inflammatory diseases like irritable bowel syndrome. [49]

In the teenage years, these same problems persist but are complicated and made worse due to the hormonal changes of adolescence and persistent social pressures. Anxiety, hormonal irregularities, and trouble sleeping are commonplace. If acne becomes embarrassing enough, antibiotics or liver-stressing dermatological drugs are voluntarily ingested, further increasing the body's chemical burden and fueling the fight-or-flight response. This is yet another vicious cycle.

In teenagers and adults, ongoing GI upset combined with regular adrenaline surges or adrenaline dominance is health-destroying. It is a guarantee. The two are inextricably linked. For this reason, the deeper GI tract is a major player in functional illness and a major focus for wholistic healers. But it all starts with the stomach, usually in the form of low stomach acid.

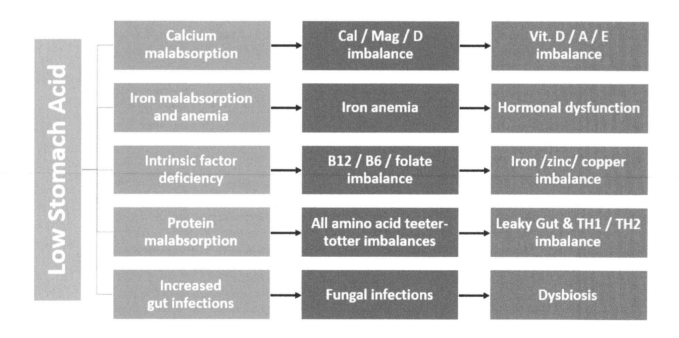

HYPOCHLORHYDRIA (LOW STOMACH ACID)

Correcting hypochlorhydria is one of the first things I do when helping a patient overcome adrenaline dominance and many other digestive issues as well. It is a necessary first step because **without appropriate levels of HCl, minerals are not properly unbound into their free form for absorption in the tissues, and proteins are not fully metabolized into their amino acid building blocks.** Skipping this step is why many people, who are otherwise making smart health choices, fail to get well.

Hydrochloric acid is the big missing piece in functional medicine. Its benefits are well known and discussed, but far too often it has been overlooked in a patient's protocol or used and then abandoned way too soon. Not only does HCl aid in the digestion of proteins and the absorption of minerals, but it also reduces the total amount of minerals needed to be ingested in the first place.

For example, the RDA for calcium is between 1200 and 2000mg per day. The RDA for potassium is 4700mg per day. Most people know that they are not getting these levels from their diet and so take a supplement (usually in the wrong form) with a full RDA's worth. In my practice, if the patient requires HCl, I do not need to recommend mineral doses at or near the RDA levels. Why? Because I have found that **HCl increases the effective absorption rate two or three-fold.**

HOW DO WE MAKE HCL?

A healthy gastrointestinal system produces about 3 to 4 quarts of HCl every day. HCl production commences in the parietal cells located in the stomach. Initially, the parietal cells are over stimulated by adrenaline surges causing HCl levels to rise. However, chronic adrenaline surges soon suppress parietal cell function and result in persistent low HCl levels.

The parietal cells also make a substance called intrinsic factor. This glycoprotein is necessary for the absorption of vitamin B12, a critical b-vitamin for energy and chemical detoxification (methylation). Consequently, people with low HCl also have low B12. This is likely why so many see benefits from a B12 injection. Furthermore, B12 is balanced on a teeter-totter with iron. So, when B12 is out of balance, iron often is as well. This scenario makes hypochlorhydria one of the major causes of anemia.

Anemia from low iron or B12 (pernicious anemia) results in many systemic health problems because it is associated with the improper formation of healthy red blood cells (RBCs). RBCs have as one of their main responsibilities, the efficient use and transport of the essential nutrient oxygen, which ends up deficient when anemia is present. Low oxygen equals low energy production and an altered metabolism. As stated above, this cascade of events all started with low stomach acid levels from adrenaline surges. In fact, looking at the chart on the previous page, the effects of low stomach acid can be directly related to almost any known illness.

The symptoms of short-term hypochlorhydria include bloating, loss of appetite, constipation or loose stools, and GI cramping. However, since digestion is critical for every function of the body, a host of other seemingly unrelated symptoms are nearly always present. Paradoxically, long-term hypochlorhydria is associated with heartburn and ulcers, two things falsely believed to be the result of excess acid.

HEARTBURN AND THE HCL PARADOX

The incidence of indigestion, "simple" heartburn, and GERD increases with age, while stomach acid levels generally decline with age. If too much acid were causing these problems, teenagers should have frequent heartburn, while Grandma and Grandpa should have much less. Of course, as everyone knows, exactly the opposite is generally true."

> *Jonathan V. Wright MD. Why Stomach Acid Is Good for You: Natural Relief from Heartburn, Indigestion, Reflux and GERD (p. 20)*

Prolonged hypochlorhydria from adrenaline surges ensures that the stomach becomes mechanically overworked from trying to do the important job of food digestion without its primary digestive resource, HCl. The result is that food, which should take 40-60 minutes to prepare for passage into the small intestine, now takes two or more hours. In this state, it is a near guarantee that the linings of the stomach will become very irritated. In time, the lower esophageal sphincter—the valve between the stomach and the esophagus—also becomes compromised, failing to remain fully closed. Now "splash back" can occur. This means the stomach contents, which are still acidic, come in contact with the tissues of the esophagus causing burning and pain.

So, it seems paradoxical, but it is true, the vast majority of those who suffer from acid reflux, GERD (Gastro-esophageal Reflux Disease) and/or ulcers, in reality, have low levels of stomach acid.

Given that acid levels naturally decline with age and that most people who have heartburn or GERD actually have low amounts of stomach acid, the push for acid-reducers is both harmful and completely backwards. Yet, it remains the first line of treatment for heartburn.

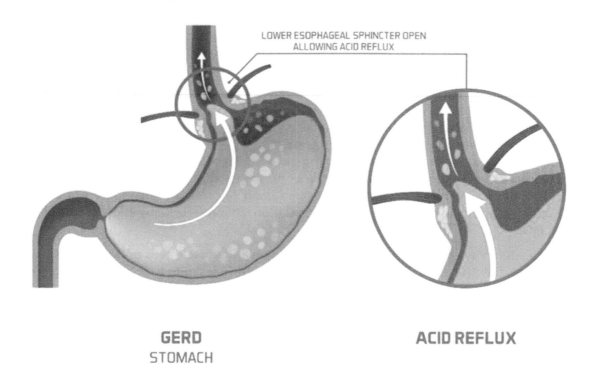

LOWER ESOPHAGEAL SPHINCTER OPEN
ALLOWING ACID REFLUX

GERD
STOMACH

ACID REFLUX

MILK AND HYPOCHLORHYDRIA

Milk and milk-based products are the number one food type to reduce stomach acid levels. This is because milk is comprised of calcium carbonate and phosphate, which together have an alkalizing effect (pH increase) making protein digestion more difficult. Milk has plenty of protein too. It also has lots of fat. Not surprisingly, HCl levels are often low in those with poor fat metabolism, gallbladder disease, or gallstones.

SHOULD HAVE ALMOND MILK INSTEAD?

The public has been brainwashed into thinking they must get their calcium from animal milk sources—"it does a body good." So, the first thing the consumer who is switching from animal to plant-based milk is going to ask is, "where am I going to get my calcium?" Not to worry. The manufacturers of almond, coconut, and other plant milks knew this and were ready with an answer. Their products proudly display a sticker that says, "50% more calcium than milk!" This sounds great, except for one giant problem. The supplemental calcium used is almost always the carbonate form. If that were not bad enough, one cup of these milks supplies forty five percent of the daily requirement for calcium or around 500 mg. This means, every cup is like drinking an antacid tablet.

THE DANGERS OF ANTACIDS

Roughly 60 million Americans experience heartburn every month.[50] While approximately 25 million Americans will suffer from peptic ulcer disease at some point in their lifetime. Each year, there are 500,000 to 850,000 new cases of peptic ulcer disease and more than one million ulcer-related hospitalizations.[51]

Over-the-counter antacids are the drug of choice for these people, making antacids one of the most used self-prescribed medications. The primary ingredients are calcium carbonate, magnesium, and aluminum salts in various combinations. The effect of antacids on the stomach is partial neutralization of gastric hydrochloric acid and inhibition of the pepsin enzyme.[52] Long-term use of antacids to lower HCl is very harmful, leading to conditions such as bone softening (osteomalacia), osteoporotic fracture, renal damage, infection (pneumonia and clostridium difficile infection), the death of muscle fibers (rhabdomyolysis), nutritional deficiencies (vitamin B12, magnesium and iron), anemia, low blood platelets (thrombocytopenia), and milk-alkali syndrome, a condition characterized by high blood calcium and metabolic alkalosis.[53]

Why is low HCl so detrimental? The main reason is that tissue and muscle cells must have free, not bound, minerals to properly function. Bound forms are stable but neutral, meaning they have little to no beneficial effect. Only when acted upon by sufficient amounts of HCl are bound minerals set free, becoming highly active. In the case of calcium specifically, not being able to make use of the bound form but still needing calcium every moment for many essential functions in the blood, cells, and tissues, the body has no choice but to extract free calcium from the bones.

DON'T EAT CHALK

To make matters worse, there are two scenarios that effectively assure osteopenia and osteoporosis will occur when HCl is chronically low. The first is by taking a few thousand international units (IU's) of vitamin D daily without taking an absorbable calcium like a citrate or malate form at the same time. The other is by taking a calcium-based antacid, which is many times consumed by those with osteopenia, believing the additional calcium will benefit their bones. Sadly, in both instances, what was meant to help, instead brought great harm. It should also be stressed that baking soda, or sodium bicarbonate, is just as alkalizing as calcium carbonate and should also be reasonably avoided.

With regards to vitamin D, this vitamin has hormone-like power and will demand and get any resources it needs to perform its functions. Stripping free, unbound calcium from the bones and teeth is often one of those resources. Calcium antacids on the other hand, are made with the most bound and hardest form of calcium to digest – calcium carbonate – aka, chalk, or limestone. Calcium carbonate is extremely alkalizing to the stomach, which, in most cases, is the exact opposite of what the body needs.

HIATAL HERNIA

Fight-or-flight chemistry directly affects the frequency of acid reflux as mentioned, but it also indirectly causes acid reflux through a condition called a hiatal hernia. Excess adrenaline leads to faster, shorter breaths and strain of the diaphragm - the muscle that contracts to allow expansion of the lungs. The diaphragm is located along the bottom of the lungs and above the stomach. To reach the stomach, the esophagus passes directly through the diaphragm. Under the influence of fight or flight, this opening begins to stretch. If this state is not changed, the apex of the stomach can peer through this opening and become pinched, resulting in a hiatal hernia. I have regularly seen hiatal hernias resolve by calming the CORE 4 and with simple in-office and at-home techniques to manually retract the stomach by applying steady and then rapid pressure in a foot ward direction.

ALKALINE WATER AND ALKALINE FOOD MYTHS

The acid-alkaline diet, the alkaline ash diet, or just the alkaline diet, is based on the idea that replacing acid-forming foods with alkaline foods can improve health. This is misguided.

The "ash" part of the alkaline ash diet comes from the idea that when things burn, an ash residue is left behind. Similarly, the foods you eat also leave an "ash" waste product behind after they are broken down and metabolized. This waste can be alkaline, neutral, or acidic. It is wrongly believed that the body's pH is directly affected by the leftover ash. If you eat foods that create an acidic ash, it makes the blood more acidic, which we are told, will make you vulnerable to illness and disease. The alkaline foods, on the other hand, "alkalize" your body and improve health.

The alkaline diet encourages a high consumption of fruits, vegetables and healthy plant foods while restricting processed junk foods. This is good. Some studies show positive effects for those with chronic kidney disease, where a low protein, "alkalizing diet" is used. This too is good. However, the alkaline diet is healthy because it is based on whole and unprocessed foods and the removal of junk foods. Doing these two things will improve health, but these benefits have nothing to do with pH levels as I will now discuss.

YOUR PH LEVEL HAPPENS NATURALLY

The letters "pH" stands for "potential of hydrogen." Hydrogen (H) is ubiquitous in the body (think H_2O), and it is also a highly acidic molecule. Adding hydrogen makes something more acidic and lowers its pH. The ranges of pH are from 0 to 14:

- **Acidic:** 0.0–6.9

- **Neutral:** 7.0

- **Alkaline (or basic):** 7.1–14.0

You can easily monitor the pH of your saliva and urine with pH paper or urine sticks. Generally, health professionals believe that both of these should be alkaline. The problem is, pH in saliva and urine changes based on your last meal, stress, lack of rest, and more—there is no set level for the pH of urine and saliva. **Blood, however, is kept in a tight pH range that, no matter what you eat, is slightly alkaline (7.36-7.44)** [54] Blood pH outside of this normal range can be fatal if left untreated. [55] But this too is related to certain disease states like ketoacidosis from diabetes and alcoholism, and therefore, has little direct influence from the diet. Only tiny fluctuations in blood pH are attributable to what is eaten daily.

Why is this so? Because the body has several effective ways to finely tune blood pH balance through a sophisticated process called acid-base homeostasis. For instance, the pancreas makes bicarbonate to control acidity in the small intestine and the kidneys allow us to urinate away many acids while producing bicarbonate ions that neutralize acids in the blood. Beyond the bicarbonate buffering system, several buffering systems are active throughout the body, like the respiratory system, which exhales acidic carbon dioxide; the hemoglobin buffer inside red blood cells; the ammonia buffer resulting from liver detoxification; the phosphate buffer within all cells; and finally, bone and certain proteins also act as buffers.

DO NOT DRINK BAKING SODA

"But I read that taking two teaspoons of baking soda helps you live longer." Actually, what you probably read, is that people who do not have enough bicarbonate in their blood and tissues do not live as long.[56] This is true. It is also true that bicarbonate is made in the body and is the vital part of its natural buffering system. Since this is a normal feature of human function, **a failure to generate bicarbonate internally is, definitionally, a sign of poor health or disease.** It is also true that bicarbonate is very alkalizing and so is sodium bicarbonate (baking soda). "So, taking baking soda is good for you then, right?" No, this is false.

The stomach is where digestion really kicks off. The acid contained within is intense, having a pH range between 2–3.5. This isn't an arbitrary level. This super acidity is necessary to break down food, especially proteins, and to absorb minerals by freeing them from their bound form. Acid does much more as well.

Acid is the first line of defense for bacterial infections, yeast overgrowth, and microbiome stability (the most common probiotic in the small intestine is acid-friendly L. acidophilus). Knowing just this so far, **does it really make sense to alkalize a system that is designed to use acid as its primary means of digestion?**

LOW BICARBONATE = LOW HCL

Trying to get bicarbonate into your body by drinking baking soda ensures that you will neutralize all the acid in your stomach. This is a terrible idea. People with low bicarbonate in their bodies already have lowered stomach acid (HCl levels). Why? Because bicarbonate and HCl are both made as products of the same process. They go hand in hand.

A LITTLE HCL CHEMISTRY

HCl is produced inside the parietal cells of the stomach using water (H_2O) and carbon dioxide (CO_2). These come together to form carbonic acid (H_2CO_3). A special enzyme called carbonic anhydrase separates carbonic acid into a hydrogen ion (H^+) and a bicarbonate ion (HCO_3^-).[57]

Now, the bicarbonate is taken from the inside of the parietal cell out to the blood in exchange for a chloride ion (Cl^-). The Cl^- then binds with the hydrogen in the stomach to make HCl. Ta Da!

So, there is a mechanism for bicarbonate to leave the parietal cell, but not one to let it back in. This means that **drinking baking soda does not transfer the bicarbonate into your bloodstream through the stomach.** When ingested, baking soda quickly reacts with the acid of the stomach, neutralizing them both. Trying to get bicarbonate into your bloodstream by ingesting baking soda or calcium carbonate is like trying to satisfy your thirst by swimming in a lake.

The physiological truth is, since HCl and bicarbonate are both made via proper function of the parietal cells, increasing bicarbonate in the blood requires making more acid in the stomach, not reducing, or neutralizing it by drinking baking soda.

Do not forget, chronic stress lowers acid levels. Therefore, HCl supplementation to restore acid levels in the stomach is one of the most common recommendations I give my patients. Taking HCl allows the parietal cells to rest and recover, just as having a soft-food diet allows the overworked stomach lining to heal.

Remember we said that HCl production starts with water and CO_2? This means that people who do not drink enough water or who do not exercise, which improves oxygen usage and CO_2 elimination, are reducing their ability to make HCl in the stomach and bicarbonate in their blood. This ignites a cascade of unhealthy reactions. Bottom line: fix your low bicarbonate by fixing your gut and acidifying your stomach, not by drinking baking soda.

CANCER AND ACIDITY

We all probably have heard of, or know someone, who was diagnosed with colon cancer, who stopped eating meat, and now is doing great. This anecdotal evidence is used as conclusive proof that meat was the cause of their cancer. Indeed, there are plenty of problems with meat quality these days and I will not argue that some of the fillers, additives, and preservatives could make it easier to contract cancer. But that is only part of the answer and is not the primary point.

Meat itself is what is being blamed—all kinds, every kind. It is blamed because meat is purported to make you acidic, and cancer grows in an acidic environment. But that is not true. Comprehensive reviews on the relationship between diet-induced acidosis and cancer conclude that there is no direct link.[58]

Remember, food does not significantly influence blood pH.[59] Even if it could, cancer cells are not restricted to acidic environments. Cancer grows in normal body tissue, which has a slightly alkaline pH of 7.4. Some tumors do grow faster in acidic environments, but it is the tumors themselves that create the acidity. This means it is not the acidic environment that creates the cancer, but the cancer that creates the acidic environment.[60]

Likewise, as I have mentioned before, there must be sufficient acid in the stomach for protein to be digested and minerals to be absorbed. If heavy meat eaters lack ample acid, then the meat they eat will putrefy in their small and large intestine creating inflammatory reactions, heavy nutritional costs, and immune system excitation. It is in this immuno-confused environment that cancer is likely to develop. Meaning, it is not a meat problem, but an undigested, putrefying meat problem.

Finally, it is hard to blame meat exclusively for cancer anyway, since those who decided to stop eating meat and had successful cancer outcomes, likely also stopped sugars, drank more water, ate more vegetables, gave up alcohol, reduced their stress, took nutritional supplements, got more rest, and started exercising. In other words, they balanced their CORE 4.

BONES AND STONES

Many alkaline-diet proponents believe that to maintain a constant blood pH, your body pulls alkaline minerals like calcium from the bones to buffer the acids from the acid-forming foods you eat. This theory is known as the "acid-ash hypothesis of osteoporosis."

I agree that osteoporosis is the result of the body pulling calcium from the bones, but it is not because the calcium is needed to buffer acids in the blood, it is because there is little useable calcium available from the diet to build and strengthen bones in the first place.

Calcium is not just calcium. It is bound to acids like carbonic acid, citric acid, malic acid, and so forth. It takes hydrochloric acid from the stomach to free calcium from what it is bound to. Adrenaline dominance suppresses acid levels in the stomach, ensuring that a bunch of bound minerals, especially calcium, are floating around in the blood wreaking havoc. The body cannot use bound calcium for its plethora of cellular functions, so it yanks free calcium from its storage sites - the bones. Now you have the mechanism for osteoporosis—not acidic foods, but an alkaline digestive tract created from an abundance of stress, CORE 4 imbalances and too many alkalizing foods like milk products.

The acid-ash hypothesis of osteoporosis fails to recognize the body's many ways to combat excess acidity and ignores one of the main drivers of osteoporosis—a loss in the protein collagen from bone. The scientific evidence linking the amount of acidic food and protein in the diet to bone density or fracture risk is mixed. This is not surprising, since it is not the protein itself that is the issue. It is whether one has enough acid in their stomach to digest the protein properly. Meanwhile, studies do show that acidic diets increase calcium retention and activate IGF-1, a hormone that stimulates the repair of muscle and bone. [61]

KIDNEY STONES

The kidneys are the body's mineral managers. They regulate the balance between sodium and water and control the concentration of many other mineral salts, such as potassium, calcium, phosphorus, and magnesium. They also help balance the pH of the body by removing waste products. An easy way to support the kidneys is to drink plenty of water—at least half a gallon per day – since most people suffering from chronic conditions are dehydrated. [62] [63]

Males are four times more likely to develop stones. Other risk factors include family history, chronic dehydration, or little fluid intake. The frequency of stones increases greatly in those with urinary tract blockage, recurring urinary infections, bowel disease, and certain inherited disorders.

There are five common types of kidney stones. By far, calcium-based stones are the most common. Calcium oxalate stones make up about 70 - 80 percent of all stone types. The remaining types are made of calcium phosphate (often mixed with calcium oxalate), struvite (related to infections), uric acid, and cystine.

The kidneys also produce specific hormones. Renin helps control blood pressure, while erythropoietin is responsible for stimulating the production of red blood cells. The decrease or absence of this hormone inevitably leads to anemia. The activated form of vitamin D, when present in the kidneys, allows the absorption of calcium and phosphorus in the intestine, making the kidneys an essential contributor to bone health.

Each of your kidneys is made up of nearly a million vascular tissues called nephrons. Kidney stones are much likelier to form when the nephrons become inflamed or scarred from excess immune chemicals, blood sugar imbalances, high blood pressure, or poor mineral breakdown. Each of these states are directly related to adrenaline dominance.

Additionally, those prone to kidney stones have low stomach acid or are people who do not do well with dairy products, both of which lead to too much bound calcium that must be eliminated. However, doctors rarely advise patients with kidney stones to stop ingesting dairy products. This is a mistake. Instead, doctors instruct their patients to avoid foods containing high oxalate levels such as spinach. To make a stone, oxalate is what bound calcium adheres to, but the answer is not to get rid of nutrient-filled spinach, but to acidify the stomach and drop the dairy.

Further proof that the problem lies with dairy and not with spinach is that even those with no familial history of stones can develop them if blood calcium rises too quickly. This happens to those who become sedentary due to illness or injury and to astronauts on long space flights, since life without gravity immediately begins to weaken bones, dumping calcium into the blood. It is excess and bound calcium in the blood that causes kidney stones to develop, not because NASA put too much spinach on the menu.

GALLSTONES

The gallbladder is a small, pear-shaped organ on the right side of the abdomen, just beneath the liver. When the gallbladder is distressed, pain can be experienced in the right upper quadrant of the abdomen, the right shoulder, and/or on the right side of the upper back. Symptoms that mimic acid reflux are also common. If any of these situations occurs, it is likely that gallstones are present.

Gallstones are hardened deposits of digestive fluids that form in the gallbladder when digestion is poor. The gallbladder holds a fluid called bile that is released into the small intestine when fat is present. Bile is a fat emulsifier aiding both in digestion and detoxification. Think of it as dish soap needed to clean a greasy pan.

HCl is crucial in stimulating proper bile production and secretion. When HCl is deficient, bile becomes thick, gallbladder function becomes sluggish, and gallstones are often created. When HCl is taken in its commonly available form, Betaine HCl, the betaine and the HCl work as a team to breakdown fats and dispose of chemicals and toxins accumulated in the liver and rest of the body. Improving gallbladder function means taking liver detoxifying products at the same time such as milk thistle, beet root, the amino acid taurine, and others.

HELICOBACTER PYLORI AND ULCERS

The normal between-meal "resting" pH level in the stomach is a 3 or less. In this environment, bacteria can live for only about fifteen minutes. As the pH rises to 5 or more, many bacterial species can survive and thrive. Without intense and regular acid baths to drive them out, the stomach can become a hospitable locale for colonization. It's dark, it's warm, it's moist, and it's often full of nutrients.[64] The stage is now set for ulcers and infections to form.

A specific bacterium, called helicobacter pylori (H. pylori) is responsible for two-thirds of all ulcers.[65] [66] The other third is mostly from NSAIDS, like ibuprofen or acetaminophen. Most H. pylori infections occur in the duodenum.[67]

H. pylori is nothing to fool around with. It is associated with coronary artery disease and arteriosclerosis.[68] Long-term H. pylori infection is directly linked to gastric cancer, the second most common cancer worldwide. In countries such as Colombia and China, H. pylori infects over half the population, beginning in childhood. In the United States, where H. pylori infection is less common in young people, gastric cancer rates have decreased since the 1930s.[69]

Nearly everyone has some level of H-Pylori in their stomach and GI tract. Although H-Pylori causes ulcers, not everyone has ulcers. Then who are the susceptible people who get a full-blown H-Pylori infection with an ulcer? Answer: those with low stomach acid, those managing prolonged stress, or those facing overwhelming stress all at once. Remember, up to one third of all ulcers come from over-consumption of NSAID drugs. People who take NSAIDS are trying to manage some sort of pain, which itself often results from the abundance of chemicals generated from the stress response or adrenaline dominance.

ACID BLOCKERS HELP ME. SO, WHY STOP THEM?

Using pharmacological acid suppression to heal peptic ulcers and to manage patients with GERD has been very successful, so much so that elective surgery for ulcer disease is now essentially non-existent.[70] The reason is because the pain induced from hydrochloric acid in contact with esophageal tissue and inside a deteriorated and inflamed stomach is quite real. Shutting down acid levels will stop this pain and allow damaged tissues to heal. So, antacids in this specific scenario are warranted. However, acid reduction alone is not the full reason for the healing. And as we have seen already, extended use of antacids causes significant systemic illnesses. Therefore, once healing has taken place, antacids should be abandoned long-term, or only used in rare circumstances.

With ulcers, antibiotics are commonly used alongside acid blockers. These halt the H-Pylori infection. Interestingly, H-Pylori infections have been shown to lower stomach acid levels.[71] This makes sense. We already know that people with high levels of stomach acid are not the ones getting H-Pylori infections because their acid level kills microorganisms and yeasts. Likewise, if acid levels rose instead of declined as H-Pylori bacteria were increasing, the whole process would be self-limiting – the infection would snuff itself out. Instead, H-Pylori thrives in low acid environments and killing it with antibiotics or herbal compounds allows acid levels to rise once again.

Another reason for ulcer recovery is the passage of time from the onset of a stressful circumstance or event. The adage, "Time heals all wounds" is true in many respects. For ulcers, the longer the acid-squelching stress is in one's rearview mirror, the more stomach acid levels can rebound.

Finally, when people get sick or have debilitating pain, they finally slow down. Their bodies simply will not allow them to do as much. This means the chemical and emotional demands from daily life are reduced as well. All of these are reasons for the eventual "healing" of an ulcer. But the absence of an ulcer does not mean that all is well. The underlying food issues and nutritional imbalances, along with persistent adrenaline surges, are still present and must be resolved.

NATURALLY HEALING HEARTBURN & ULCERS

As we have learned, high acid is rarely the issue with heartburn. Instead, increasing acid levels, avoiding alkalizing substances, and taking steps to heal a damaged stomach lining are the proper route to take. Foods that irritate, alkalize, or promote intestinal yeast overgrowth, must also be avoided.

Some people cannot tolerate much HCl at first. This is because there is simply too much tissue damage in the stomach. For those people, apple cider vinegar is a less potent but helpful option, so long as they do not have intestinal or vaginal yeast problems. At the same time, until HCl can be added without issue, herbal products that heal the stomach and those that kill infections are used.

Natural remedies are often just as effective as antibiotics for H-Pylori infections and do not have the side effects that antibiotic use can bring. Flavonoids from plants,[72] the mineral bismuth citrate, marshmallow root, slippery elm root, berberine, and deglycyrrhizinated licorice root (DGL),[73] when used in combination, can all help heal ulcers, kill H. pylori, and repair the stomach lining at the same time.[74]

These supplements will need to be taken for several months along with those required to calm adrenaline dominance. All the dietary steps and details to heal heartburn and dozens of other digestive issues are presented in STEP 3: the *Gentle GI Diet*.

THE BRAIN AND IRRITABLE BOWEL

Your central nervous system (CNS) is your brain and spinal cord. The CNS constantly receives information via your five senses: visual stimulation from your eyes, touch sensation from your skin, sound from your ears, gravitational input to your joints and muscles, taste from your tongue, and smell from your nose.

Just as regular physical exercise keeps muscles strong, the constant stimulation by our senses through the nerves up the spinal cord and into the neurons keeps the brain alert and active.

There is so much information coming into the brain at any given moment, that if we had to pay attention to all of it, nothing would ever get done. Therefore, ninety percent of the brain's responses to stimuli are subconscious and involuntary. Only ten percent are volitional.

For instance, if a fly lands on your ear at a social event, you can reflexively jerk your whole body while swatting wildly into the air and run the risk of being disruptively convulsive, or you could consciously override the urge by swishing away the pesky invader with a smooth unnoticed motion of your hand. In this scenario, YOU HAVE VOLUNTARY CONTROL.

The other ninety percent of your brain's output includes activities such as digestion, heart rate, and respiration. These functions are running 24/7 WITHOUT OUR CONSCIOUS AWARENESS. This means that one of the best ways to have a healthy gut is to have a healthy brain. Amazingly, it also goes the other way around.

The enteric nervous system (ENS), also known as the intrinsic nervous system, is embedded throughout the linings of the gut from the esophagus to the anus and governs the function of the entire GI tract. The interaction between the ENS and brain is often described as THE GUT-BRAIN AXIS and has been sparking the interest of researchers for many years.

Traditionally, neurotransmitters and neuromodulators were thought to function only in the central nervous system. However, it is now believed that these chemicals influence a wide range of activities throughout the body. [75]

IBS AND THE BRAIN

Ninety percent of the important neurotransmitter, serotonin, is found within the ENS. This is perhaps a major mechanism by which the activity in the gut microbiome directly messages the brain. Behavior, mood, and cognition are all related to this gut-to-brain communication. Unintentionally, depression treatments targeting serotonin levels in the brain will negatively impact the gut and sometimes to a strong degree. Irritable bowel syndrome (IBS), for instance, afflicts more than two million Americans and arises in part from too much serotonin in the gut. It is therefore, a "mental illness" of the second brain. [76]

HCL AND THE VAGUS NERVE

Remember how important hydrochloric acid is for the digestion of proteins and the absorption of minerals? The vagus nerve (aka cranial nerve 10) is the direct path from the brain to the gut. One of its jobs is to activate the stomach's parietal cells for the release of HCl. However, a tired, inflamed, or otherwise unhealthy brain, results in an unhealthy nervous system and improper activation. Of course, there are many other CORE 4 imbalances to consider, but improper nerve impulse transmission through the vagus nerve is another possible mechanism where brain degeneration can lead to poor digestion and absorption.

EMOTIONS AND THE GUT

All emotions have a direct relationship to a particular organ. The emotion most related to stomach irritation is anxiety. Pressure situations, such as public speaking or doing anything significant for the first time, can cause "butterflies in the stomach." We are all familiar with this sensation just prior to participating in an anxiety-producing event. The "stress" of the experience causes adrenaline to surge, the sympathetic nervous system to ramp up, and the stomach to shut down. In the long-term, this means a significant drop in hydrochloric acid levels (hypochlorhydria) and the creation of a vicious chemical cycle:

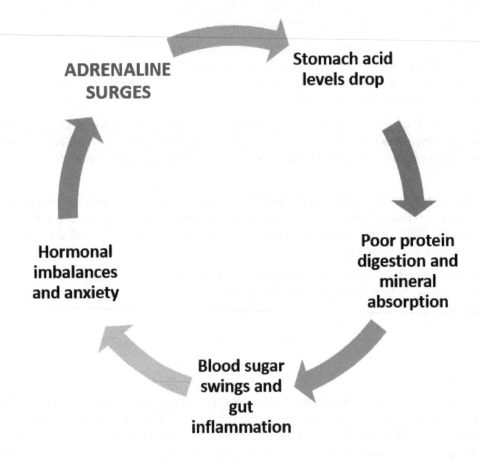

THE MICROBIOME

The healthy human intestine is colonized by over 1000 types of bacteria forming a microbial ecosystem called the gut flora, microbiota, or microbiome. Over 100-trillion individual organisms composing nearly five pounds-worth commensal bacteria, engage in a network of cooperation and competition.

Most of the microbiome is located in the small intestine, a 30-foot-long section of the digestive tract located between the stomach and the large intestine, is where enzymes, acids, and good bacteria all work together to break down fats, proteins, and carbohydrates into their smallest parts. The body then uses these raw materials for the growth, repair, and fuel for all cells and systems. The yeoman's work of digestion takes place here.

Based on importance and function, the microbiome could easily be considered another vital organ within the human body. It helps regulate a wide variety of physiological processes such as b-vitamin formation, regulation of mood, cognition, and even pain, which are all part of the gut-brain axis. In fact, the microbiome can affect nearly every aspect of life. The levels of neurotransmitters are greater in the gut than the brain by a factor of nine, making the microbiome part of the "second brain."

A clearer picture is emerging of the composition of the human microbiome and its balance in healthy individuals. A normal gut microbiome can generate colonization-resistance, meaning it prevents the overgrowth of disease-causing gut pathogens. Disturbances of the microbiome via antibiotics, medications, adrenaline surges, poor diet, or a variety of diseases, shifts the inner balance. Now, opportunistic invaders can over-populate, the immune system can over-activate, and infections with inflammatory responses will likely demonstrate.

THE MICROBIOME IS PART OF THE IMMUNE SYSTEM

The relationship between the immune system and the microbiome is intimate. Loss of proper immune system communication and host control over the gut flora leads to bacterial "blooming." The significance of these interactions is particularly evident in Crohn's disease (CD) and Ulcerative Colitis (UC), whose symptoms are caused by an excessive immune response against one's own beneficial flora. Persistent adrenaline surges effect immune regulation of the gut and lower intestinal acidity from the stomach creating an environment of abnormally composed microbiota referred to as "dysbiosis." **Dysbiosis is both a cause and a consequence of inflammatory bowel disease (IBD), Type 2 diabetes, obesity, allergies, colorectal cancer, as well as less debilitating issues like gas, bloating, and constipation.** [77]

Whenever the immune system does its work of fighting off infections or cleaning up cellular debris, the result is always some level of inflammation. In a healthy immune system, the levels of inflammation go undetected and unnoticed in daily life. This is not the case when the immune system becomes unbalanced. In this state, a forest fire of pain and swelling can ignite. When inflammation is high in the digestive tract, a host of undesirable consequences emerge, the worst of which is a condition known as *Leaky Gut Syndrome*.

LEAKY GUT SYNDROME

Decades of ingesting refined sugars, bad fats, and processed foods—the 'sweets and grease' of the Standard American Diet—will inevitably lead to functional problems of all kinds. The lining of the small intestine simply cannot withstand this toxic barrage indefinitely. With every bite of processed food, the immune system increases its activity, ramping up its output of macrophages, phagocytes, and eosinophils, which are the cells responsible for cleaning up the mess. As the response increases, it challenges the stability of the small intestine. Ultimately, the lining transforms for the worse. What was once a tightly knit cellular wall allowing only selected items to move past, now contains gaping holes through which entire proteins pass directly into the blood stream.

Proteins leaking, or translocating, into the bloodstream causes a further burst of immune system activity. Antibodies form and attach themselves indiscriminately to everything that comes down the pipe. This means that people with a "leaky gut" are often allergic to a majority of what they eat. Even the simplest foods, like brown rice and green vegetables, can cause severe bloating and abdominal pain.

Leaky Gut Syndrome is the slippery slope of functional illness. If left unattended, digestive trouble will soon spill over, causing strain on the liver, kidneys, and bladder. These are the detoxification organs responsible for cleaning up the waste products of digestion. With an inflamed small intestine, they must now work around the clock to eliminate the massive load of chemical waste products produced by the restless immune system, promoting a state of autointoxication.

Signs of poor detoxification will always manifest in those with an inflamed digestive tract. Allergies, chemical sensitivities, digestive complaints of all kinds, headaches, brain fog, memory loss, and fatigue are all common.

Chemicals, both from normal metabolic processes and from the diet, create free radicals through oxidation. This constant bombardment drains the body of the important antioxidant glutathione. Once its levels are depleted the tissue-destroying agent iNOS (a form of nitric oxide) runs rampant. Its presence is directly related to Leaky Gut Syndrome and autoimmune disease.

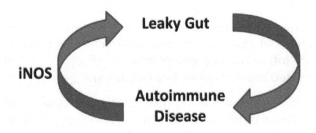

From the standpoint of hormetic nutrients, Leaky Gut Syndrome often leads to several mineral deficiencies, including magnesium, zinc, copper, calcium, boron, silicon, and manganese. Even if these minerals are high in the diet, they may not be getting to their target tissues. The inflamed linings of the small intestine disrupt the normal attachment of a mineral to its carrier protein—the taxi that drives the mineral to the cell hotel. Abandoned minerals, therefore, never make it out of the gut or into the cells. **For instance, fibromyalgia patients, those with chronic whole-body pain and fatigue, consistently demonstrate low red blood cell magnesium even with high magnesium consumption through diet and supplementation.**

Once the gut becomes leaky, just taking deficient minerals will not be enough to help. The gut wall must first be healed. Herbs such as slippery elm bark,[lxxviii] marshmallow root,[lxxix] and deglycyrrhizinated licorice[lxxx] gently repair the mucosal linings of the small intestine. These are the same products used to heal the stomach lining in those with low HCl.

The diet needed to heal Leaky Gut Syndrome is the same diet I recommend to most of my patients no matter what their ailments. This is because the gut is never not involved in functional illness. But it is inflamed, tired, and susceptible to the erratic swings of the immune and blood sugar systems. To address these issues all at the same time I use a mostly cooked vegetable, protein-based, low-grain, no dairy, no processed sugar approach for three weeks that I call, the *Gentle GI Diet* – elucidated fully in PART 3.

PARASITES

A parasite is an organism that lives on or in a host. Over 100 different types of parasitic worms can live in the human body. They range from microscopic in size to many feet long. Female worms can release 3,000 to 200,000 eggs per day depending on their type. Symptoms can range from uncomfortable to life threatening.

Parasites have been linked to almost every illness. Chronic parasitic infections drain the body of critical resources and destabilize the immune system. They can lead to secondary viral, bacterial, or fungal infections as well. Most people are living with parasites, unaware that the organisms are chipping away at their vitality. A healthy, strong immune system can and does eliminate most of these. However, if functional illness is already rampant, parasites may take up permanent residence.

Parasitic infections used to be thought of as the dread of the tropical regions. Actually, parasites live over much of the earth. Now, however, with worldwide travel being commonplace, parasites easily spread to different areas. Nationally reportable parasitic diseases tract infectious cases of these parasites: Cryptosporidiosis, Cyclosporiasis, Giardiasis, Malaria, and Trichinellosis.

TREATING PARASITES

Some parasitic diseases are easily treated, and some are not. A whole-person approach is essential to make the immune system and all other systems as optimal as possible. However, just balancing vitamins and minerals is often not enough with a strong infection. Powerful herbs like wormwood,[lxxxi] black walnut hull,[lxxxii] or Coptis Chinensis[lxxxiii] are often required.

Additionally, parasites develop through various stages and life cycles, making them harder to kill. Whichever herbal remedy is selected, it should be used for up to several months, depending on the overall severity of the infection and overall health of the patient. This consistent dose will ensure that any developing parasites are eliminated as they mature.

HORMONES

No woman or teenage boy on earth needs a doctor to tell them that reproductive hormones are powerful. These specialized proteins are responsible for a large percentage of the chemical reactions taking place in the body at any given moment.

Hormones also exemplify the interconnectedness between the systems of the body, since most hormonal imbalances come with an array of multi-organ symptoms such as:

- Blood sugar swings
- Breast tenderness
- Depression
- Edema
- Endometriosis
- Fibrocystic breasts
- Hot flashes
- Infertility
- Irregular menstrual cycles
- Loss of libido
- Osteoporosis
- PMS
- Poly Cystic Ovarian Syndrome
- Unexplained weight gain [84]
- Uterine fibroids

Hormonal disruptions will result from any CORE 4 imbalance. Things like adrenal or thyroid gland dysfunction, liver congestion, allergic reactions, fungal and other microbial infections, birth control pills, poor diet, and toxicity from environmental causes, such as pesticides and plastics.

ADRENALINE IS A THIEF

There are only so many resources to go around. For this reason, adrenaline surges have an immediate negative impact on reproductive hormones. Remember, the chemistry produced from the fight-or-flight response is meant for survival. Everything is dedicated to this task. Making babies and digesting a nice meal are not done when the grizzly bear is sniffing around outside the tent. Instead, the hormonal resources allocated to reproduction and digestion are shunted to the adrenal glands and the central nervous system for maximum adrenaline production.

Looking at the hormonal pathway on the next page and observing all the arrows pointing in different directions, gives an indication of the complexity of the hormonal system. Any one of these arrows represents a place where a breakdown can occur. The body relies on precise hormetic nutrients at these same locations to keep the hormones flowing correctly.

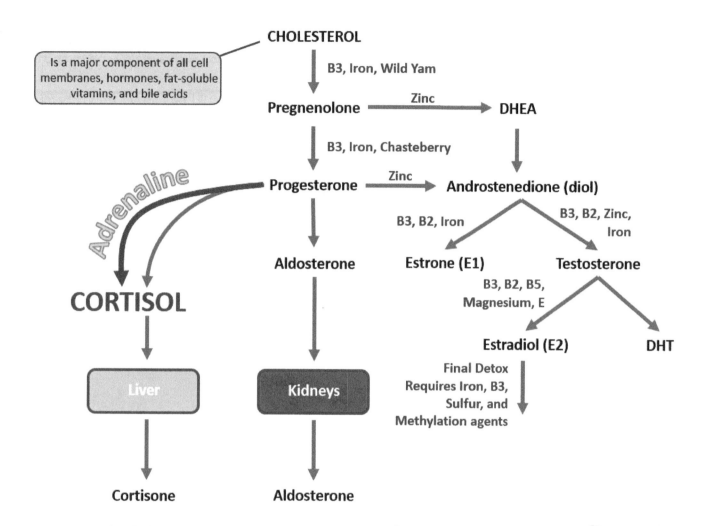

THE FEMALE SEXUAL CYCLE

The menstrual cycle should be a rhythmic cycle lasting between 20 and 45 days, with an optimal cycle lasting 28 days. Its purpose is to prepare a female's egg (ovum) for fertilization with a male's sperm and to prepare the uterus to receive and sustain the fertilized egg.

Although there is variation with the normal length of the cycle, there should be certain trends before, during, and after ovulation. For instance, if a woman experiences unpleasant symptoms, such as uterine cramping, headaches, or bloating prior to ovulation, there is likely an issue with the hormone progesterone, which surges at these times. However, if a woman experiences the symptoms just prior to menstrual bleeding, estrogen imbalances are a stronger consideration.

There are three different hierarchies of hormones to consider when discussing the female sexual cycle. The first comes from the hypothalamus and is the gonadotropin-releasing hormone (GnRH). Its job is to stimulate the anterior portion of the pituitary gland—the gland in charge of overseeing the entire cycle. The anterior pituitary gland releases two important hormones: follicle stimulating hormone (FSH) and luteinizing hormone (LH). These two then act directly on the ovaries, encouraging them to secrete estrogen and progesterone, respectively.

Day one is the first day of menstrual bleeding, but this day is also the end of some very important steps, as seen in the following graph.

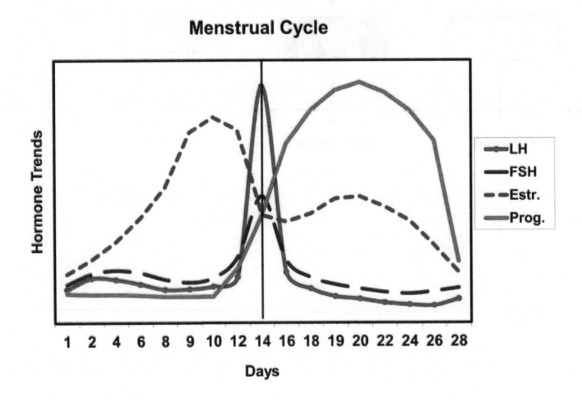

Synopsis

- Day 1: Shedding of uterine lining with increases in estrogen from days 1 through 12.

- Day 12: Marked increase in FSH, drastic increase in LH, and estrogen at its peak.

- Day 13: Dramatic drop in estrogen initiates ovulation.

- Day 14: Ovulation, FSH and LH at their peak, and progesterone rising.

- Day 13: Surge in progesterone until day 23.

- Day 15: Drop in FSH and LH.

- Day 23: Progesterone at its peak.

- Day 24: Drop in progesterone until day 28.

- Day 28: lowest levels of progesterone initiates the shedding of the uterine lining (menstrual bleeding), and the cycle repeats.

OVULATION

Ovulation is the moment when one ovary releases an egg. At birth, a woman has around one million eggs in both ovaries. Each month, after the onset of puberty, an egg contest begins. The body allows 6 to 12 eggs to participate in the contest, but only one is the winner.

Under the influence of follicle stimulating hormone (FSH), a follicle will contain each contestant. One follicle will become dominant and cause the others to die off (become atretic). Thus, the winner—the sole remaining follicle— will mature and eventually burst at the time of ovulation, releasing the egg within, now called an ovum.

For a woman with a 28-day cycle, ovulation occurs 14 days after the onset of menstruation. The first part of a woman's sexual cycle may vary from month to month by a few days. However, the last half of the cycle, from the time of ovulation to just before the start of menses, is usually a consistent 14 days. There are five characteristics of ovulation:

1. The rapid growth of the follicle by FSH.

2. Decreasing amounts of estrogen.

3. Increasing amounts of progesterone to promote pregnancy.

4. Release of the egg from the follicle.

5. A surge of LH to produce a corpus luteum.

CORPUS LUTEUM

After ovulation, the winning egg receives her crown. A cloud of granulosa cells, called a *corona radiata*, surrounds the ovum. LH, which aids in implantation, surges 6 to 10-fold two days before ovulation, transforming the granulosa cells into lutein cells. The corpus luteum is the combination of the ovum and the lutein cells. Over the next 6 to 12 days, the corpus luteum will grow, secreting progesterone and some estrogen while awaiting fertilization. If none occurs, the estrogen secretions soon shut off both LH and FSH, and the corpus luteum involutes or dies.

ESTROGEN

This is perhaps the most talked about hormone in the female cycle. It is responsible for the sexual characteristics of the female and causes the proliferation of many reproductive cells. Its job during the sexual cycle is to prepare the ovum for fertilization. Estrogen is high during the early part of the cycle and drops at ovulation. Too much estrogen is sometimes a cause for failed conception or can result in a failure to ovulate.

One of the most common gynecological problems is irregular menstrual cycles. Skipping periods, heavy bleeding, and spotting are all menstrual irregularities. When estrogen levels are high, the lining of the uterus builds up in an exaggerated manner. This overproduction leads to a dramatic release of tissue at the time of menstruation, and results in heavy bleeding.

Too much estrogen is usually associated with cramping, a shorter cycle, and a longer period. Higher progesterone levels, on the other hand, usually mean light bleeding with little pain, a shorter period, and a longer cycle.

When the overall levels of estrogen are low, the uterine lining never properly forms and frequent release, or spotting, is likely. Too little estrogen can result in vaginal dryness and hot flashes during menopause.

PROGESTERONE "PRO GESTATION"

Progesterone is the hormone most responsible for the healthy development of a baby. Many women who have trouble maintaining a pregnancy usually need to increase progesterone. Its functions during the sexual cycle include raising body temperature (incubation), preparing the uterus for pregnancy and the breasts for lactation, and inhibiting FSH and LH.

If fertilization does not occur, progesterone drops, initiating menstrual bleeding due to the shedding of the uterine lining. If fertilization does occur, then a hormone called human chorionic gonadotropin (HCG) prevents progesterone from decreasing. HCG is the hormone detected in a pregnancy test. With fertilization, HCG will be present in the urine and blood stream around one week after ovulation.

THE PITUITARY GLAND: HOT, COLD, OR RESISTANT?

A small tissue bundle on the bottom side of the brain called the pituitary gland regulates most hormones. To keep them at proper levels, the body makes hormones based upon a negative feedback loop. For instance, if a woman is low in estrogen, the pituitary gland in the brain will release another hormone called follicle stimulating hormone (FSH), which will stimulate the adrenal glands and the ovaries and encourage them to make more estrogen. If her estrogen is too high, the pituitary stops releasing FSH, and estrogen naturally drops as it is metabolized in the liver. Negative feedback loops are the teeter-totters of entire systems of the body. They are also common in everyday life.

When the house gets too cold, the thermostat "tells" the furnace to start working. Once the house is warm, the thermostat stops speaking, and the furnace no longer makes any heat. The house is similar to the human body: the thermostat is the pituitary gland, and hormones are the heat.

A healthy pituitary gland is constantly turning on and off, regulating the hormonal system in a steady, rhythmic fashion. Wild swings in hormones are a big stress for this tiny gland. Too little hormone in the body for too long means the pituitary is working overtime, while too much hormone for long periods means the pituitary doesn't work enough. This straightforward feedback of hormone regulation is beautiful in design and function, but it is also somewhat fragile and easily pushed around by adrenaline surges. There are three common patterns of functional disturbance related to the hormonal system.

PITUITARY SLUMBER – THE HORMONE HOUSE IS TOO COLD

Pituitary slumber is a regular occurrence resulting from eating too many refined sweeteners. Sugary foods cause surges of insulin. This has a drugging effect and lulls the pituitary to sleep as the body tries to manage a sweet-food surplus. Cortisol from the adrenal glands soon follows to counterbalance the high insulin levels and further suppresses pituitary function. In this state, the pituitary gland does not respond by stimulating endocrine tissues when hormones are low. Poor hormonal rhythm and blood sugar swings are the consequence.

As we continue, you will see that Insulin, cortisol, adrenaline, and white sugar are some of the most common pituitary irritants. A pattern emerges where under stress, cortisol and adrenaline increase causing a person to crave sweets. When ingested regularly (usually in the form of white sugar), the result is glucose spikes and insulin surges, followed eventually by the development of hypoglycemia and/or insulin resistance and the triggering of additional adrenaline. The vicious combination is self-perpetuating, leading to further pituitary suppression, and a massively dysregulated hormonal system. All this is the environment where PMS and migraines manifest.

PITUITARY SUPPRESSION – THE HOUSE IS TOO HOT

If the house is always hot, the thermostat never needs to tell the furnace to make heat. This may not matter to the inanimate thermostat, but it matters greatly to living tissue like the pituitary gland. Use it or lose it applies here. If the pituitary gland is not regularly involved in life's rhythmic processes, it loses tone and begins to atrophy. This happens when there is too much hormone available.

Once the body makes something, it must use it or break it down. For hormones, this is mostly the responsibility of the liver. Beginning in adolescence and encouraged by a sweets-and-grease diet, poor liver detoxification leads to excess hormone levels, especially in young women. **PMS symptoms including cramps, breast tenderness, irritability, excessive flow, and headaches, are directly related to the incomplete metabolism and breakdown of estrogen (primarily), progesterone, or one of their subtypes.** The entire process is further agitated by the unwarranted and prolonged use of birth control pills, which are usually an artificial form of estrogen (more on this topic in a moment)

Bio-identical hormone replacement therapy (HRT) is the second method that creates excess hormone and causes a state of pituitary suppression. This condition of hormonal abundance guarantees that the house becomes too hot, leading to a suppressed pituitary gland. Doctors often prescribe HRT when hormone levels in the body are low, as when women are in menopause or perimenopause. HRT is like using space heaters when the furnace is broken. This is an appropriate short-term usage. However, space heaters are not under the influence of the thermostat and leaving them on all night can be uncomfortable or even dangerous. Long-term use of hormone replacement leads to a dependence upon artificial hormone regulation and promotes a nasty situation called hormone resistance.

HORMONE RESISTANCE

Have you ever had the experience of getting back into your car after running an errand, turning the key, and immediately having the maxed-out radio blast your ears? Just a little while earlier, when a favorite song was playing, you cranked up the volume and jammed along, doing your best driver's seat dance moves. The sounds didn't shock you then, so what happened? You adapted. When the sounds were loud, the nerves in your ears re-adjusted themselves to manage the high decibels. When you went into the store, they adapted again to the less intense background sounds. However, back in the car, being instantly re-transported to the front row of the *Taylor Swift* concert, was just too much. This type of adaptation in the nervous system is called homotropic modulation. In the hormones it is called hormone resistance.

Hormones change how a cell's receptors function. If a cell is constantly bombarded by hormones, its receptor sites become over stimulated. This is an unhealthy state for the cell and the body as a whole. The receptor sites where hormones attach are like the cell's ears that hear and respond to numerous hormonal commands. Too many hormones, like too much talking at the same time, soon becomes a bothersome noise. To protect against this state, cells do what they must and close their own ears.

People experiencing hormonal resistance are in bad shape. They have too many hormones talking, but no one is listening. To further complicate the matter, in the state of hormone resistance, too much of a hormone produces the exact same outward symptoms as too little. For example, someone with hormone resistance who has too much serotonin may still suffer from depression in the same way as someone with too little. Even though the necessary serotonin is present, the body is not responding to it because it is overwhelmed with excess bombardment. It has gone deaf. Treating a patient based solely upon their symptoms will often mean prescribing a medicine or nutrient for one state, when the body may need exactly the opposite.

PMS AND ESTROGEN EXCESS

Researchers who study PMS estimate that as many as 20-30 percent of women suffer from this condition at some point in their lives. Bloating, acne, pain, emotional changes (moodiness, anger, depression), and fatigue are some of the common symptoms of PMS. Technically, to have PMS, the symptoms must occur at the same time each month. For example, if a patient's symptoms relate to high progesterone, the symptoms would occur at ovulation, near the middle of the cycle. Most PMS symptoms, however, relate to excess estrogen and would therefore occur prior to menstrual bleeding.

Attacks can also worsen when hormone levels rise or fall either after giving birth or in the transition into menopause. Migraine symptoms are generally less frequent and intense during the last six months of pregnancy. This is the teeter-totter effect in action—progesterone upsurges during pregnancy ease the symptoms of excess estrogen.

CAUSES OF ESTROGEN EXCESS

1. **ADRENALINE SURGES** — This is a powerful disrupter of hormonal balance and leads to a myriad of unwanted effects such as weight gain, sleep disruptions, adrenal gland fatigue, osteoporosis, and more.

2. **POOR DIET** — A poor diet composed of refined and processed foods disrupts digestion, leading to inflammation of the small intestine lining. This irritation then causes poor absorption of nutrients (leaky gut syndrome). Poor absorption of nutrients, in turn, eventually leads to inadequate resources for the breakdown and processing of hormones and promotes the overgrowth of unwanted organisms such as Candida.

3. **PLASTIC AND PESTICIDES (XENOESTROGENS)** — Plastics and pesticides that are absorbed into our bodies act like estrogens. In lakes with large amounts of pesticides, fish become hermaphroditic, newborn alligators are all female, and the male alligators become feminized.

4. **MEATS AND MILK** — These are another source of exogenous hormonal compounds with estrogen-like qualities. Annually, around 750,000 cows received injections of bovine growth hormone and antibiotics. Ranches often use pesticide-laden, genetically modified feed for cattle, which can have an estrogen-like effect.

5. **LIVER CONGESTION** – The liver is the organ that does all the breaking down of used hormones. If the liver is congested (full, fatigued, overworked), it likely lacks the necessary resources to detoxify female hormones. As a result, the excess hormones continue to float freely in the blood stream, interacting with estrogen receptors on various tissues and creating a hormonal overload.

6. **FUNGAL INFECTIONS** — There is a strong relationship between fungal infections and estrogen imbalances. Fungus, like Candida Albicans, thrive in estrogen-dominant women, altering the rhythmic estrogen fluctuations throughout the cycle.

7. **ADRENAL FATIGUE** — The adrenal glands are a secondary producer of estrogen. Messages from the pituitary gland force the adrenals to make more when needed. However, tired adrenals that are responding to fight-or-flight stimuli, cannot meet the demand, so the ovaries work overtime. This will result in more peaks and valleys for estrogen.

8. **ALLERGIES** — Allergens generate numerous amounts of immune system chemicals, increase inflammation in the tissues, and increase water retention and bloating, all of which make detoxification of the reproductive hormones by the liver more difficult.

9. **MEDICATIONS** — Birth control pills, hormone replacement therapy (HRT), and excess use of antibiotics, all designed to correct imbalances, often create many of their own.

10. **NUTRITIONAL IMBALANCES** — Proper quality and quantity of nutrients must be present for detoxification to take place effectively.

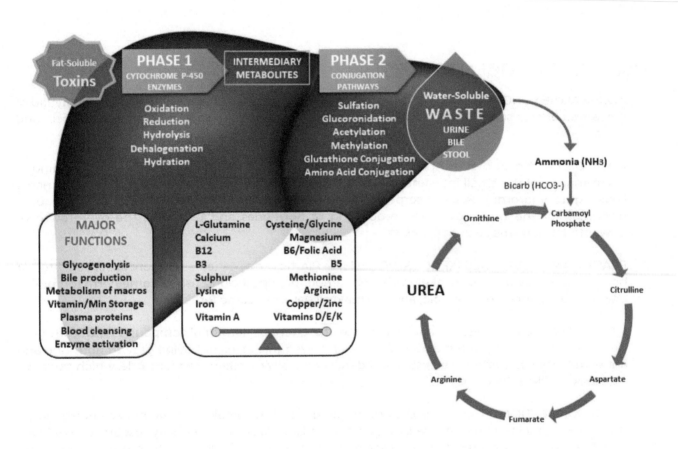

LIVER DETOXIFICATION

PCOS AND INSULIN RESISTANCE

One of the best examples of how CORE 4 Imbalances interact with and against each other to greatly disrupt the hormonal system is polycystic ovarian syndrome (PCOS), which affects 15% of women and girls of reproductive age.

Women with PCOS usually have at least two of the following three conditions: [85]

- Absence of ovulation, leading to irregular menstrual periods or no periods at all.

- High levels of androgens (male hormones like testosterone) or signs of high androgens, such as having excess body or facial hair.

- Cysts (fluid-filled sacs) on one or both ovaries—"polycystic" means "having many cysts."

PCOS often causes several other problems as well, such as unwanted hair growth, dark patches of skin, acne, weight gain, and irregular bleeding.

THE OVARIES

The ovaries are responsible for the production of female reproductive hormones like estrogen. The ovaries also make androgens, just not at the same levels as men. Ovarian cysts, however, primarily result from progesterone, whose job is to stimulate the ovaries at ovulation to promote the release of an egg. The failure of egg-release called anovulation, initiates even greater hormonal response from progesterone. This bombardment of stimuli alters the structure of the ovaries causing the follicles—small, fluid-filled cysts within the ovaries in which eggs grow and mature—to enlarge, forming cysts.

Despite plenty of functional imbalances, many women do not know they have PCOS until they have trouble getting pregnant. This is because PCOS is the most common cause of anovulatory infertility, meaning that an egg failed to release at the time of ovulation.

INSULIN RESISTANCE

Insulin resistance is the primary reason for the disordered hormonal status of those with PCOS. It is the job of insulin to transport glucose into the cells. High carbohydrate diets overload the body with glucose, and consequently high insulin, to manage the glucose. This abundance of insulin begins to desensitize the cells to its presence, making them resistant to insulin's knock on the cellular door. High levels of insulin can also increase appetite and lead to weight gain, while in some thickened, dark skin, called acanthosis nigricans, appears.

Too much insulin increases the production of male hormones, especially testosterone, which then turns around and blocks the receptor sites for insulin on the cells, creating a vicious cycle. In women, the additional testosterone also leads to excess facial hair and thinning hair on the scalp. It also alters estrogen and progesterone levels, affecting neurotransmitter activity in the brain. Drive, motivation, and personality can be altered as well. And lastly, testosterone interferes with the normal brain signaling that initiates ovulation, so that ovulation becomes irregular.

The combination of blood sugar and hormonal imbalances in women with PCOS is why they are also at risk for:

- Obstructive sleep apnea, a disorder that causes pauses in breathing during sleep.

- Metabolic syndrome, a group of risk factors for heart disease and type 2 diabetes.

- Type 2 diabetes

- Obesity

- Heart disease and high blood pressure

- Mood disorders

- Endometrial hyperplasia, a condition in which the lining of the uterus becomes too thick, and endometrial cancer.

HRT AND BIRTH CONTROL PILLS

Many books have been written espousing the benefits of hormone replacement therapy (HRT) to keep the body young, strong, and wrinkle-free. The practice of giving replacement hormones when they are low in the body is, on the surface, logically sound. However, digging a little deeper reveals a few potential problems.

In July of 2002, the National Institutes of Health (NIH) halted a large, in-progress, study examining the effects of a widely used type of HRT medication called Prempro,® which combines the hormones estrogen and progestin. The NIH took action because the hormones increased a woman's risk of breast cancer, as well as heart disease, blood clots, and stroke. The findings were published in *JAMA*, the Journal of the American Medical Association.

A review of preliminary data found a 26 percent increase in breast cancer, a 29 percent increase in heart attacks, and a 22 percent increase in total cardiovascular disease among women receiving the hormones compared with women who received a placebo. Three months later, a British HRT study was also stopped for essentially the same reasons. There had been hopes HRT could reduce the risk of coronary heart disease, but the reverse appears to be true.

These results are not at all surprising to many operating in the realm of natural medicine. In fact, doctors have known for almost 30 years that estrogen replacement by itself increased the likelihood of some cancers. That is why both aborted studies above combined artificial progesterone (progestin) along with estrogen. Even this combination together was not enough to prevent significant side effects.

Proponents of HRT use compounds consisting of non-synthetic, bio-identical hormones like the ones made within the body. This is reasonable. When the body requires hormones, it needs natural hormones— not synthetic versions. However, there is more to the story.

Natural hormone replacement can be very useful in some instances, such as after a hysterectomy, thyroidectomy, or other surgeries that require the removal of hormone-producing tissue. HRT may also be appropriate when an autoimmune or congenital disease has damaged hormonal tissues, when exhausted hormone-regulating glands need a short-term break, or in menopause or perimenopause. In these cases, a doctor must regularly monitor the replacement hormones to prevent hormone resistance from hormone excess.

BIRTH CONTROL PILLS

Every week I treat young women for a host of complaints related to hormonal imbalances and adrenaline surges. Many of them, because of painful, heavy, or headache-making menstrual cycles, opted sometime in the past to take a birth control pill as recommended by their MD. Often, their horrible monthly symptoms improved, so it must have been a good thing, right? Perhaps.

If the young woman will not stop eating her low-protein, sugar, and chocolate-filled diet; not go to bed before midnight; not drink water, or not put down the stress-creating, brain-numbing phone, then yes, putting her on a pill to artificially alter the most basic and fundamental cycle of womanhood might be the best thing to do. Everything in life is based on the choices we make.

From a natural perspective, however, disregarding the hormonal sensitivity within the endocrine system, its intricate arrangements, impressive power over metabolism, mood, memory and more, is to also disregard the magnificent inter-connectedness of the body, and essentially to live for the next moment of instant gratification and not for long-term health (ugh...I'm glad I got that off my chest).

I use strong language around the topic of hormones and young ladies for a few reasons. First, I am the father of five daughters, all of whom are different physically and emotionally and none of whom has had any symptomatic reason (difficult PMS) to ever consider taking the birth control pill. If some PMS symptom should arise, they all have been trained to know it is because of a food they have over consumed, a lifestyle choice they have adopted, or a specific supplement they need. Second, In the case of adolescent hormonal management, the contrast between allopathic and natural medicine could not be more stark. Likewise, in this instance the slogan of natural physicians who exclaim that they are *looking to find and remove the root cause, helping the body do what it was designed to, while allopathic doctors simply cover up symptoms with medications, creating other problems in the process,* is entirely true. Third, correcting hormones in young woman using the approaches taught here is not difficult, is easy to implement, and is regularly "miraculous."

Given the number of hormonal issues that plague women throughout their lives—ovarian cysts, fibroid tumors, endometriosis, infertility, PCOS, depression, hypothyroidism, insomnia, etc.—getting them balanced when they are young and teaching them to maintain their balance is true healthcare.

THE NEGATIVE EFFECTS OF BIRTH CONTROL PILLS

Birth control pills are one of two types. The first type keeps estrogen high so the follicle-stimulating hormone and luteinizing hormone peaks do not happen. This prevents an egg from developing properly or prevents ovulation altogether. The second type keeps progesterone high so the body thinks it is pregnant, thereby not releasing additional eggs. Both cause hormone resistance—estrogen resistance in the former case, and progesterone resistance in the latter—neither of which is ever a good long-term solution. Hormone resistance can....

- lead to excessive uterine bleeding, blood clots, hypertension, depression, vomiting, increased weight, kidney disease, and ovarian atrophy,

- confuse the body's natural hormonal production, which in the very least will eventually make menopause difficult,

- create fibroid tumors. Thankfully, fibroid tumors oftentimes spontaneously go away at menopause because of a drop in estrogen,

- lower vitamin B6 levels, which can lead to depression, food allergies, carpal tunnel syndrome, and sensitivities to electromagnetic fields,

- negatively affect fertility after disuse,

- result in recurrent yeast infections.

When told about the negative effects of birth control, women are often shocked and reply, "My doctor never told me that!" If a woman feels the need to use birth control pills at this time in her life, then, at a minimum, she should work with a health professional capable of monitoring the effects of the synthetic hormones and who will support her therapeutically in whichever ways most effectively help to minimize the detrimental consequences.

MIGRAINES AND THEIR CAUSE

Migraine headaches affect more than 30 million Americans, including 10 percent of children. According to the National Headache Foundation (NHF), 70 to 80 percent of migraine sufferers have a family history of migraines.

A migraine is a severe, debilitating form of headache that typically appears as a throbbing ache near the side of the forehead and can last in some cases up to one week.

There are well-known triggers for migraines and other clues that help define its cause of action and reason for recurrence.

- Women have migraines three times more often than men. [86]

- 75 percent of women get migraines at ovulation or near the start of their cycle. [87]

- Migraines affect up to 37 percent of reproductive-age women, the time when most women are menstruating. [88]

- Common triggers of migraines include noise, light, hormonal changes, sleep disturbances, stress, intensive physical activity, and foods such as chocolate, red wine, cheeses, processed meats, the preservative MSG, caffeine, and alcohol (food issues often mean trouble with liver detoxification).

As we have discussed already, the reproductive hormone estrogen (and often progesterone) are a trigger with most migraines. However, other hormones are involved, as well. The fight-or-flight response, which induces high levels of cortisol and adrenaline, often triggers a migraine. So can insulin when released because of blood sugar swings. Each of these chemicals has the potential to initiate a migraine, but only if the hormonal environment in the brain is out of balance.

THE PRIMARY IMBALANCE: DOPAMINE AND SEROTONIN

Researchers know that migraines are a vascular headache in nature because of the direct involvement of the blood vessels in the brain. During a migraine, vascular tissues swell allowing greater blood flow. The reason this happens is because a migraine is the brain's emergency means to rapidly remove excess neurotransmitters (brain hormones), so they do not overstimulate the nervous system and impair proper cerebral function. But which neurotransmitters? There are two. Serotonin and dopamine.

Dopamine is by far the least provocative of the two but will cause a migraine under the right conditions. For example, if someone begins to treat extreme sleepiness from narcolepsy, shift work sleep disorder, or obstructive sleep apnea by taking a central nervous system stimulator like Provigil, they could experience a migraine. This medication directly activates the dopamine receptor sites. Too much however, creates excess excitation of these receptors and triggers a protective vascular response from the brain to "dilute" the chemistry, aka a migraine.

Dopamine involvement, in my estimation, is only responsible for around 10-15% of all migraines. Serotonin is by far the primary hormonal troublemaker. This is confirmed by the medications used for migraine pain relief. Maxalt (Rizatriptan Benzoate) can reduce many migraines in just minutes. It does this by constricting the blood vessels and by directly blocking the receptors sites related to serotonin, making it act like less serotonin is present. [89]

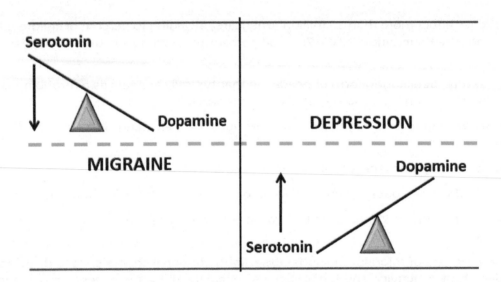

Serotonin is powerfully impactful on a slew of bodily functions, which is why it is closely regulated by the brain. But, second only to the blood sugar system, the serotonin pathway may be the most susceptible to damage from the effects of emotional stress.[90][91] When serotonin is too low, it causes depression—when its levels are too high, migraines can result.

The solution to migraine resolution is to make sure the hormetic nutrients used to metabolize or "lower" serotonin are present in ample amounts. The question then becomes, "why were those nutrients deficient in the first place?"

Looking back to the discussion in Part 1: The cause of nearly all functional illnesses comes from CORE 4 imbalances set on fire by adrenaline dominance. This means what is required to eliminate migraines and balance hormones is a whole-person, CORE 4-balancing approach as described in PART 2: *The 50 FIX Plan*.

As stated throughout, reducing stress and adrenaline dominance is essential and must be intentional. Likewise, for the sake of health, a person should consider lifestyle choices, career paths, peripheral relationships, and commitments of all types based upon the amount of emotional and physical stress likely to be generated. The new "busy" is simply far too busy. The body has its limits and many in the modern have exceeded those limits (see STEP 9: *Relocate*).

MIGRAINES AND ANTI-DEPRESSANTS

Serotonin as a medication is well-known for its role in helping people with depression. The cost of depression and other mental illnesses is nearly 300 billion dollars annually. Over seven million women in the United States have clinical depression, according to the National Mental Health Association. Women are twice as likely as men to suffer from depression, indicating a strong hormonal connection to the problem. In fact, estrogen (primarily its estradiol form) strongly influences the serotonin receptors in the brain, increasing or decreasing their sensitivity.

About 10 percent of Americans, or 30 million people, are currently taking anti-depressants. That number is double what it was only a decade earlier and has shown no signs of slowing down. [92] [93]

The type of medication most taken for depression is an SSRI, or a selective serotonin reuptake inhibitor. It is the job of these medications to prevent the body from processing serotonin, thus keeping its levels high in the brain. The result is people with low serotonin feel better. This sounds good, but it is not without significant problems. Re-uptake prevention will certainly ensure that plenty of serotonin remains in the brain. **However, this can be a strong trigger for migraines.** Also, downstream substances like melatonin—a popular sleep helper—may end up deficient since serotonin is not being metabolized fully. This is perhaps why so many people taking anti-depressants also need to take sleep aids at the same time. Remember, serotonin is but one step in a sophisticated and somewhat fragile pathway (shown on next page).

The overall effectiveness and safety of SSRIs has come under scrutiny in recent years. Scientists at Duke University Medical Center tested exercise against the drug Zoloft and found the ability of either, or a combination of the two, to reduce or eliminate symptoms was about the same percentage. However, exercise alone seemed to do a better job of keeping symptoms from coming back after the depression lifted. Their findings, reported in the *Journal of Psychosomatic Medicine*, suggest a modest exercise program "is an effective, robust treatment for patients with major depression." [94]

Beyond the effectiveness question, anti-depressants have a darker side, as well. Prolonged use of anti-depressants can suppress immune function, [95] [96] effect sexual function [97] and may even promote suicide. [98]

The above findings are not surprising since, from a neurological point of view, depression results from low firing of the frontal cortex, which body movement from exercise and brain stimulation from new mental challenges can improve. Also, as a matter of physiology, SSRIs do not and cannot fix broken neurotransmitter pathways. Thankfully, hormetic nutrients and improved CORE 4 balance can.

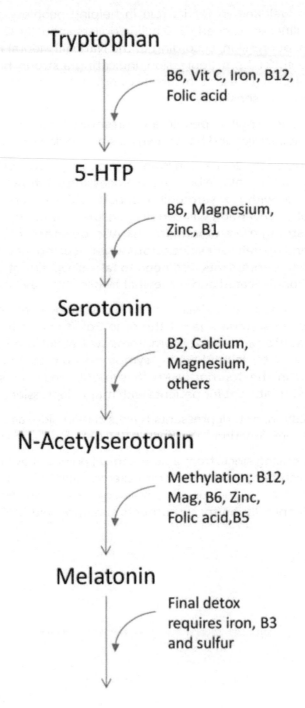

Tryptophan

B6, Vit C, Iron, B12, Folic acid

5-HTP

B6, Magnesium, Zinc, B1

Serotonin

B2, Calcium, Magnesium, others

N-Acetylserotonin

Methylation: B12, Mag, B6, Zinc, Folic acid,B5

Melatonin

Final detox requires iron, B3 and sulfur

LOW ESTROGEN AND THE BRAIN

With PMS and migraine, the goal is to reduce elevated and poorly metabolized estrogen. However, the estrogen suite of hormones is powerful and extraordinarily helpful. Without sufficient estrogens brain inflammation and degeneration are increased through the following actions:

- Reduced inhibition of the self-perpetuated stress response, making the brain hyper-reactive to even mild stress triggers.
- Failure to dampen activated immune cells (microglia) in the brain, leading to inflammation.
- Increased circulating immune chemicals, called cytokines, cause inflammation, and increases their total number of receptors and the sensitivity of those receptors.
- Lowered ability to make glutathione, the most powerful antioxidant in the body.
- Altered good fatty acid balance toward, regardless of diet, toward a pro-inflammatory state.
- Decreased bone marrow activity, raising the risk of osteoporosis, a disease with a strong inflammatory component.
- Slowed healing of the lining of the GI tract and the blood-brain barrier (leaky gut and leaky brain).

These factors explain why menopause brings on so many distressing symptoms and why it raises the risk of certain inflammatory and degenerative conditions such as heart disease, stroke, arthritis, certain autoimmune diseases, osteoporosis, dementia, and Alzheimer's. Sadly, for the perimenopausal and menopausal woman, just raising estrogen levels may not be enough. Studies show that even after estrogen levels are restored, the inflammatory cytokines (immune system chemicals) continue to stay upregulated. Meaning that estrogen replacement alone was insufficient to halt brain inflammation. Complete CORE 4 rebalancing with the *50 FIX Plan* is required to help tame adrenaline and the myriad of other rogue inflammatory substances.

IMMUNE SYSTEM

Currently, humanity is experiencing the longest life spans since the time of Moses. And yet, the rates of cancer, heart disease, obesity, and diabetes are also at their highest levels. How is it possible that these two facts can be true at the same time? The answer is modern medicine's and modern society's greatest achievement—microbial management – the elimination of bacteria, viruses, and other disease-promoting microorganisms.

For the splendid work accomplished in the areas of disease control, the scientists of medicine and sanitation deserve the praise of all. Because of their achievements in microbial management, plagues are less of a concern today although some scares remain. Presently microbes are less often a threat to life in 1st world countries but are still a threat to health and full human function.

Even if an organism is not directly involved in a disease, its mere presence still requires an immune system response, which results in a continual drain on the body's nutritional resources. Therefore, if the immune system can manage, quarantine, or kill the microorganisms, there is a good chance to maintain health and extend longevity.

THE IMMUNE SYSTEM: HOW IT WORKS

An incredibly complex defensive network, called the immune system, is the body's main form of resistance against various stressors. Nearly 60 percent of all immune system cells are in the linings of the intestines. A person's greatest exposure to the outside world is through the food he eats, which may be full of harmful chemicals or bacteria. This is one reason people with chronic illnesses and weakened immune systems almost always have digestive complaints at the same time.

The immune system works aggressively to promote healing and tissue repair after injury and to eliminate dead cells and improperly developing cells (cancer). The bulk of the immune system, located within the linings of the small and large intestine, is the Gut Associated Lymphoid Tissue (GALT). The linings of the nose, mouth, throat, and lungs contain another web of immune tissues, called the Bronchus Associated Lymphoid Tissue (BALT). Besides these areas, the organs most responsible for immune system support and function are the bone marrow, thymus, spleen, and liver.

LEUKOCYTES

White blood cells, called leukocytes, are the cells that increase in number when the body is trying to fight a new (acute) infection. There are several types of white blood cells, each with specific immune-related functions: neutrophils, eosinophils, basophils, monocytes, and lymphocytes. For the purpose of a general immune system overview, the focus shall remain on the last type, the lymphocyte, and its role in fighting unwanted antigens and haptens.

ANTIGENS AND HAPTANS

Antigens and haptens are any substances that, when present, generate an immune system response. Examples of antigens include bacteria, viruses, and foreign proteins. Haptens are inorganic, or non-living, things consisting of heavy metals, pesticides, chemicals, etc. The chart below demonstrates the basics of what occurs when an antigen or hapten appears in the body.

The first response by the immune system is to "tag" or mark, any undesirable substance for destruction or elimination. This is the job of the antigen-present cells (APC). Next, the APC sends out specific chemical messengers, called cytokines, which call other important "helper" cells to the scene to eliminate the antigen.

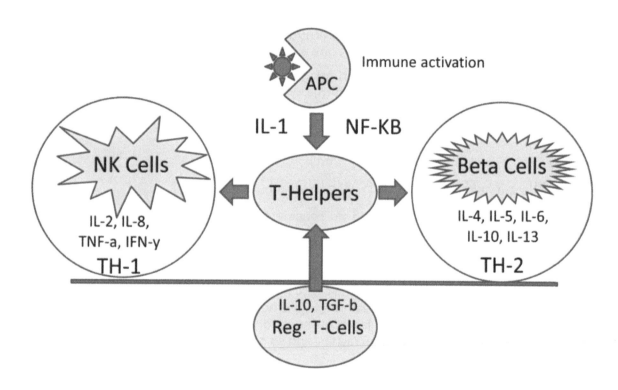

Once the process is underway, the immune system can basically follow two paths, called the TH-1 path or the TH-2 path. The TH-1 path supports the production of natural killer cells (NK cells). The TH-2 path promotes Beta cells (β-cells). In the early stages of antigen destruction, the immune system relies mostly on NK cells. If the infection is strong or lasts for a long time, then it will place more emphasis on the production of β-cells.

The β-cells make people "immune" to things by producing antibodies. For instance, if a person had the chicken pox as a child, then she most likely will have chicken pox antibodies in her blood, which ensures that she will no longer get that condition in adulthood. This individual has become immune to the chicken pox.

After the immune system eliminates the antigen, it must turn off the cytokines. Otherwise, there will be a continuous signal for help. There is no need for more wood on the fire when the house is already hot. It is the business of the Regulatory T-cells and the Suppressor T-cells to shut down the immune system when it finishes the job. When all goes well, the antigen is eliminated, cytokines are no longer produced, and the body is now free from invasion/infection. Unfortunately, chronic illness often means the house is either way too hot or it ran out of wood long ago. Either way, the environment is quite uncomfortable.

Before chronic illnesses set in, functional imbalances from adrenaline dominance were taking their toll on the body and altering the normal feedback loops from the immune system. Now the body must make a choice. Keep fighting, or adapt? It is common for seemingly "normal" or "healthy" people to be in a state of adaptation.

Adaptation simply means the body is using resources from one area to support the deficits of another. Constant adaptation comes at great expense. Eventually, the reserves and tissues responsible for continuing the adaptation process fatigue and finally fail. Like a leaky roof left untended, significant future damage is certain.

TILTING OUT OF BALANCE

Immune system imbalances are no laughing matter. When a dysregulated immune system is present, just about any symptom could result. Worse yet, autoimmune diseases, multiple chemical sensitivities (MCS), Chronic Fatigue, Fibromyalgia, or hypothyroidism are a long-term likelihood.

For instance, a survey of 1,582 respondents from Atlanta, Georgia found that 12.6 percent reported MCS. The prevalence for this condition is similar in California, where the Department of Health Services reported 15.9 percent, and suggests the national prevalence may be similar.[99] This number is more than double what it was in the year 2000.

THE IMMUNE SYSTEM CAUSES WEIRD STUFF

There is a debate as to whether MCS should be considered a diagnoseable condition. This is not too surprising since traditional medicine is so compartmentalized and MCS results from many CORE 4 imbalances all at the same time.

From my perspective, I have seen onions cause debilitating arthritic reactions; the wrong supplements cause recurrent yeast infections; microorganisms cause lower back pain; chocolate cause debilitating hip and neck pain; an old ankle injury cause ear ringing; emotional stress cause carpal tunnel; handling dandelions cause immediate and massive leg bruising; and yes, exposure to everyday chemicals cause headaches, depression, extreme fatigue, skin rashes, and so on. There is no debate for me.

AUTOIMMUNE DISEASE

Approximately one in five people suffer from autoimmune disease,[100] which is the process whereby one's immune system attacks its own tissues. Autoimmunity is a special threat to women, whose prevalence is three times that of men. Autoimmune disease is among the ten leading causes of death for women in all age groups up to 65.[101]

The type of autoimmune disease a person has depends on its location. Rheumatoid Arthritis (RA) affects the joints, Multiple Sclerosis (MS) targets the sheath around the nerves, Type I Diabetes Mellitus affects the pancreas, Crohn's disease attacks the small intestine, and Hashimoto's affects the thyroid gland. These are just a sample of the more than 80 illnesses caused by autoimmunity.

WHERE DOES AUTOIMMUNE DISEASE COME FROM?

One could make a compelling case that microbes such as bacteria, viruses, fungi, and parasites, are the cause for autoimmune disease. Rarely, if ever, will a health professional find a condition unrelated to bugs to some extent. For instance, heart disease in some is directly linked to burrowing bacteria called helicobacter pylori.[102] [103] The primary cause for hypothyroidism in America is autoimmune thyroid or Hashimoto's. This process of thyroid self-destruction is many times initiated by a virus.[104] Diabetes directly connects to imbalances between the "good" and "bad" bacteria in the digestive tract.[105] [106] Arthritis may in fact relate to a deep-seated infection.[107] Cancer, many believe, results from poor gene expression, which has direct ties to the constant assault of microorganisms, such as the human papilloma virus and its relationship to cervical cancer.[108] Additionally, researchers are investigating the association between breast cancer and three other viruses,[109] one of which is the Epstein-Barr virus, the cause of mononucleosis, which is a common ailment among teenage girls.[110]

Beyond microbes, researchers around the world search for environmental, genetic, hormonal, and nutritional clues without much success. Perhaps their thinking is too specialized? Adrenaline dominance is a whole-body imbalance resulting in many functional illnesses all at the same time.

Is there still a hidden infection in the gut or mouth? Is the patient full of heavy metals? Has the person eaten foods that the digestive system cannot breakdown or that the liver cannot detoxify? Is there improper genetic expression because of nutritional deficiencies? Is fight-or-flight raging? Autoimmune diseases have no single cause. They are the result of many imbalances that facilitate and promote other existing imbalances. They are the ultimate expression of a perfect CORE 4 storm.

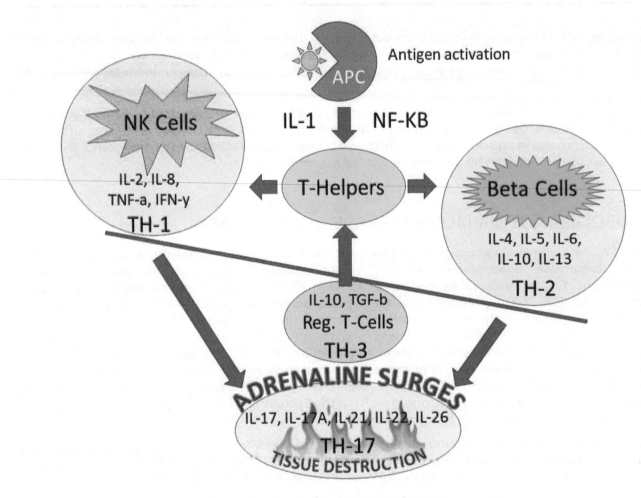

The Teetering Immune System

TEETERED IMMUNE SYSTEM

The most common immune dysregulation is an imbalance between the two types of helper cells, TH-1 and TH-2. Often there is an overabundance of immune system activity within one of these categories and not enough with the other. Here again is an example of one of the body's many teeter-totters. Most asthma patients, for instance, have a great deal of TH-2 activity, whereas TH-1 activity is often too high in those with Multiple Sclerosis.

When the immune system is teetering, an increase in a group of cytokines, collectively called TH-17, occurs and inflammation erupts. The result is ongoing tissue damage like what is seen in the autoimmune skin condition psoriasis.[111]

The way to regulate this imbalance is threefold. First, the side that is too active needs to be dampened. This often means removing agents that stoke the immune system's fire. Second, the side that is too low needs to be stimulated. This is done with specific nutraceuticals and hormetic nutrients. Finally, the brake in the middle of the teeter-totter needs to be firmly applied. These are the regulatory and suppressor cells of the TH-3 system. Immune modulators, such as vitamin D, glutathione, and healthy oils are the brakes.

WHICH NUTRIENTS HELP AUTOIMMUNITY?

To help autoimmunity, the trick is to know which side to stimulate...TH-1 or TH-2? Here are some common nutritional supportive agents that I recommend for balancing the autoimmune teeter-totter. There is just one problem...none of them will work. None will work, that is, if you do not do the entire *50 FIX Plan*. Autoimmunity is a 24/7 disease and requires an all-hands-on-deck approach. No exceptions. You can do it!

- TH-1 function too low – increase it with substances you would take if you had a cold like echinacea, zinc, and astragulus.

- TH-2 function too low – increase it with substances like green tea, berberine, artemisia, white willow, and grape seed extract.

- TH-1 or TH-2 function too high – detoxify the immune chemicals (cytokines) that continue to signal for help. This is done primarily by supporting the liver.

- Hit the brakes – To stimulate immune system modulation via the regulatory cells (TH-3) add Vitamin D, EPA, DHA, and/or glutathione.

PART 4: THE FUNCTIONAL HEALTH ASSESSMENT (FHA)

Before you can get to where you want to go, you must first know where you are. The FHA has nine categories with fifteen questions each. To complete the test simply circle "yes" if the question applies to you. The circled answers are then added together and converted into a grade value that can be superimposed on the *Stress Threshold* graph. Repeat this test every six weeks as you employ the strategies described in the *50 FIX Guidebook,* and watch your grade improve!

Part 1, Blood Sugar Imbalances

	Date _____	Date _____	Date _____
Always hungry?	Yes	Yes	Yes
Brain fog after eating?	Yes	Yes	Yes
Buzzing or shaking in hands, intermittent?	Yes	Yes	Yes
Crave sweets after meals?	Yes	Yes	Yes
Depressed mood that is helped by sweets?	Yes	Yes	Yes
Eat something sweet before bed often?	Yes	Yes	Yes
Energy drops in the afternoon?	Yes	Yes	Yes
Fatigue after eating breads or carbohydrates?	Yes	Yes	Yes
Headaches with exertion or stress?	Yes	Yes	Yes
Not hungry in the morning?	Yes	Yes	Yes
Numbness in toes or fingers not related to injury?	Yes	Yes	Yes
Shaky, lightheaded, or irritable with missed meals?	Yes	Yes	Yes
Skip breakfast often?	Yes	Yes	Yes
Sugar makes you feel good?	Yes	Yes	Yes
Urinating more than once per night?	Yes	Yes	Yes
TOTAL	_____	_____	_____

Part 2, Brain Strain

	Date	Date	Date
Can't remember the names of people you just met?	Yes	Yes	Yes
Difficulty calculating numbers?	Yes	Yes	Yes
Feel disinterested with former hobbies?	Yes	Yes	Yes
Feel hopeless about my situation?	Yes	Yes	Yes
Feel little compassion for others?	Yes	Yes	Yes
Feel that life is meaningless?	Yes	Yes	Yes
Feel uninterested with life?	Yes	Yes	Yes
Feel you have no purpose?	Yes	Yes	Yes
Feelings of dread or impending doom?	Yes	Yes	Yes
Lack of mental focus causes poor problem resolution?	Yes	Yes	Yes
Hard time finishing tasks?	Yes	Yes	Yes
Hobbies and interests are few or none?	Yes	Yes	Yes
Loss of long-term memory?	Yes	Yes	Yes
Mind often wanders while doing important things?	Yes	Yes	Yes
Short-term memory loss?	Yes	Yes	Yes

TOTAL _____   _____   _____

Part 3, Upper Gut Imbalances

	Date	Date	Date
Acid reflux?	Yes	Yes	Yes
Asthma past or present?	Yes	Yes	Yes
Coated or fuzzy tongue?	Yes	Yes	Yes
Food allergies?	Yes	Yes	Yes
Food sensitivities (non-gluten)?	Yes	Yes	Yes
Fungus under finger or toenails?	Yes	Yes	Yes
Gluten sensitivity?	Yes	Yes	Yes
Hair becoming finer?	Yes	Yes	Yes
Heartburn?	Yes	Yes	Yes
Kidney stones?	Yes	Yes	Yes
Muscle cramps (Charley Horse)?	Yes	Yes	Yes
Nails are weak, have ridges, or peel?	Yes	Yes	Yes
Regular burping after meals?	Yes	Yes	Yes
Stomach aches?	Yes	Yes	Yes
Stomach ulcers?	Yes	Yes	Yes

TOTAL _____ _____ _____

Part 4, Lower Gut Imbalances

	Date	Date	Date
Abdominal bloating after eating?	Yes	Yes	Yes
Abdominal pain?	Yes	Yes	Yes
Antibiotics more than three times in life?	Yes	Yes	Yes
Bad breath often?	Yes	Yes	Yes
Constipation often?	Yes	Yes	Yes
Diarrhea after a fatty meal?	Yes	Yes	Yes
Diarrhea often?	Yes	Yes	Yes
Gallstones?	Yes	Yes	Yes
Generally have digestive complaints or upset?	Yes	Yes	Yes
Hemorrhoids often?	Yes	Yes	Yes
Lower back pain?	Yes	Yes	Yes
Nasal or sinus congestion?	Yes	Yes	Yes
Spider veins?	Yes	Yes	Yes
Spoon-shaped indented nails?	Yes	Yes	Yes
Varicose veins?	Yes	Yes	Yes

TOTAL _____ _____ _____

Part 5, Hormonal Imbalances

	Date _____	Date _____	Date _____
Excessive hair loss?	Yes	Yes	Yes
Facial hair growth?	Yes	Yes	Yes
Headaches often?	Yes	Yes	Yes
Hot flashes?	Yes	Yes	Yes
Irregular monthly cycles?	Yes	Yes	Yes
Migraine headaches?	Yes	Yes	Yes
More than 10 pounds overweight?	Yes	Yes	Yes
Night sweats?	Yes	Yes	Yes
Outer third of eyebrow thinning?	Yes	Yes	Yes
PMS (emotional, or cramping, or breast tenderness?)	Yes	Yes	Yes
Sexual desire or performance, loss of?	Yes	Yes	Yes
Skin, wrinkling rapidly?	Yes	Yes	Yes
Sun exposure less than 15 min. per day?	Yes	Yes	Yes
Trouble losing weight even with exercise?	Yes	Yes	Yes
Vision changes throughout the day?	Yes	Yes	Yes

TOTAL _____ _____ _____

Part 6, Immune System Imbalances

	Date	Date	Date
Arthritis (under age 50) or autoimmune disease?	Yes	Yes	Yes
Catch colds easily?	Yes	Yes	Yes
COVID 19 caused severe symptoms?	Yes	Yes	Yes
Eczema or psoriasis?	Yes	Yes	Yes
Feel worse in humid, damp, or moldy places?	Yes	Yes	Yes
Loss of taste or smell?	Yes	Yes	Yes
Muscle tenderness without exercise?	Yes	Yes	Yes
Pain or swelling in joints?	Yes	Yes	Yes
Pet or environmental allergies?	Yes	Yes	Yes
Prostatitis or vaginitis/yeast infections?	Yes	Yes	Yes
Rashes or hives?	Yes	Yes	Yes
Ringing in ears?	Yes	Yes	Yes
Sickness requiring antibiotics once a year or more?	Yes	Yes	Yes
Slow healing sores?	Yes	Yes	Yes
Steroids needed for immune system or pain relief?	Yes	Yes	Yes

TOTAL _____ _____ _____

Part 7, Nutrient Imbalances

	Date _____	Date _____	Date _____
Drenching sweat with exercise?	Yes	Yes	Yes
Dry skin?	Yes	Yes	Yes
Fatigue that is not from lack of sleep?	Yes	Yes	Yes
Growing pains as a child?	Yes	Yes	Yes
Heart palpitations?	Yes	Yes	Yes
Heel spurs?	Yes	Yes	Yes
High blood pressure?	Yes	Yes	Yes
Muscle tightness or inflexibility generally?	Yes	Yes	Yes
Neck pain not from trauma?	Yes	Yes	Yes
Pins and needles in arms not from trauma?	Yes	Yes	Yes
Plantar fasciitis?	Yes	Yes	Yes
Poor night vision?	Yes	Yes	Yes
Restless legs?	Yes	Yes	Yes
Swelling in ankles?	Yes	Yes	Yes
Visual floaters in eyes?	Yes	Yes	Yes

TOTAL _____ _____ _____

Part 8, Adrenal Gland Imbalances

	Date	Date	Date
	_____	_____	_____
Anxious often or for no apparent reason?	Yes	Yes	Yes
Can't turn off my mind when it is time to relax?	Yes	Yes	Yes
Chest pains from anxiety?	Yes	Yes	Yes
Cold hands or feet?	Yes	Yes	Yes
Crave salt?	Yes	Yes	Yes
Caffeine required to get going?	Yes	Yes	Yes
Caffeine make you feel bad or jittery?	Yes	Yes	Yes
Dizzy or lightheaded upon standing?	Yes	Yes	Yes
Less than 8 hours of sleep per night?	Yes	Yes	Yes
Light bothers eyes (always wear sunglasses)?	Yes	Yes	Yes
Shortness of breath?	Yes	Yes	Yes
Sweaty hands and feet?	Yes	Yes	Yes
Trouble falling or staying asleep?	Yes	Yes	Yes
Under frequent high stress?	Yes	Yes	Yes
Weight loss without diet or lifestyle changes?	Yes	Yes	Yes

TOTAL _____ _____ _____

Part 9, Detoxification Imbalances

	Date	Date	Date
Acne on face?	Yes	Yes	Yes
Acne on back or legs?	Yes	Yes	Yes
Alcohol/wine bothers in low doses?	Yes	Yes	Yes
Burning pains on skin?	Yes	Yes	Yes
Cold sores?	Yes	Yes	Yes
Drink less than 5 glasses of water per day?	Yes	Yes	Yes
Electronics or EMFs cause issues?	Yes	Yes	Yes
Exercise causes brain fog or sickness?	Yes	Yes	Yes
Gout or Hepatitis?	Yes	Yes	Yes
Itchy skin not from dryness?	Yes	Yes	Yes
Pains around or under the rib cage?	Yes	Yes	Yes
Skin reactions to jewelry?	Yes	Yes	Yes
Strong smells cause irritation or symptoms?	Yes	Yes	Yes
Taking daily medication(s)	Yes	Yes	Yes
Water retention or puffiness often?	Yes	Yes	Yes

TOTAL _____ _____ _____

FINISHED!

You have completed the *Functional Health Assessment*.
Now it is time to calculate your score and letter grade.

To calculate an overall health grade, add up the total number of "Yes" answers. Once you have the sections added together, find the corresponding grade on the chart below.

GRADE	TOTAL SCORE	FUNCTIONAL COMPLAINTS
A	<15	FEW
B	16-30	LOW TO MODERATE
C	31-50	MODERATE
D	51-65	ELEVATED
F	>65	EXCESSIVE

Now, match the grade with the corresponding letter on the *Stress Threshold* graph below. This is your current placement.

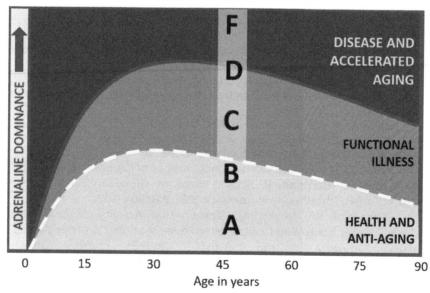

If your results did not turn out so great, this is not too surprising. Functional illnesses are why you picked up and began reading this guidebook. Many patients started from a troublesome spot just like you, but now they have an A or a B grade because they followed the 10 STEPS of the *50 FIX Plan*. Now it is your turn. Flip back to PART 2 and get started!

REFERENCES

[1] Buford TW, Willoughby DS. Impact of DHEA(S) and Cortisol on Immune Function in Aging: A Brief Review. Appl Physiol Nutr Metab. 2008 Jun;33(3):429-33.

[2] Fontana L. Neuroendocrine Factors in the Regulation of Inflammation: Excessive Adiposity and Calorie Restriction. Exp Gerontol. 2009 Jan-Feb;44(1-2):41-5.

[3] Van Santen A, Vreeburg SA, et al. Psychological Traits and the Cortisol Awakening Response: Results from the Netherlands Study of Depression and Anxiety. Psychoneuroendocrinology. 2010 Aug 17.

[4] Mujica-Parodi LR, Renelique R, Taylor MK. Higher Body Fat Percentage is Associated with Increased Cortisol Reactivity and Impaired Cognitive Resilience in Response to Acute Emotional Stress. Int J Obes (Lond). 2009 Jan;33(1):157-65.

[5] Thau L, Gandhi J, Sharma S. Physiology, Cortisol. [Updated 2022 Aug 29]. In: StatPearls [Internet]. Treasure Island (FL): StatPearls Publishing; 2022 Jan-. Available from: https://www.ncbi.nlm.nih.gov/books/NBK538239/

[6] Graham, Danielle. Genetics, Epigenetics and Destiny. An Interview With Bruce Lipton. http://www.superconsciousness.com

[7] ND., Ben Lynch. Dirty Genes (p. 2). HarperOne. Kindle Edition.

[8] U.S. Department of Health and Human Services. (2003). National Survey of Child and Adolescent Well-Being: One Year in Foster Care Wave 1 Data Analysis Report. Retrieved April 27, 2006, from www.acf.hhs.gov/programs/opre/abuse_neglect/nscaw/reports/nscaw_oyfc/oyfc_title.html

[9] Kelley, B. T., Thornberry, T. P., & Smith, C. A. (1997).In the Wake of Childhood Maltreatment. Washington, DC: National Institute of Justice. Retrieved April 27, 2006

[10] English, D. J., Widom, C. S., & Brandford, C. (2004). Another Look at the Effects of Child Abuse.*NIJ journal*, 251, 23-24.

[11] Long-Term Consequences of Child Abuse and Neglect www.childwelfare.gov/pubs/factsheets/long_term_consequences.cfm#societ

[12] https://ct.counseling.org/2018/10/the-storm-and-stress-of-adolescence-and-young-adulthood/

[13] https://www.cdc.gov/healthcommunication/toolstemplates/entertainmented/tips/SuicideYouth.html

[14] https://www.niddk.nih.gov/health-information/health-statistics/overweight-obesity

[15] Flegal K, Carroll M, et al. **Prevalence and Trends in Obesity Among US Adults, 1999-2008**. *JAMA*. 2010;303(3):235-241.

[16] https://health.usnews.com/health-news/blogs/eat-run/2015/06/11/think-youre-sensitive-to-gluten-think-again

[17] Kharrazian, Datis. Why Isn't My Brain Working?: A revolutionary understanding of brain decline and effective strategies to recover your brain's health . Elephant Press.

[18] http://www.mypyramid.gov/STEPS/stepstoahealthierweight.html

[19] https://www.nih.gov/news-events/nih-research-matters/how-too-little-potassium-may-contribute-cardiovascular-disease

[20] https://www.ncbi.nlm.nih.gov/pmc/articles/PMC3417219/

[21] Schmitt, Walter H. Compiled Notes on Clinical Nutrition Products; 1990. p. 46

[22] https://www.ncbi.nlm.nih.gov/pmc/articles/PMC4848870/

[23] Setnikar I, Giacchetti C, and Zanolo G. Pharmacokinetics of Glucosamine. *Drug Res* 1986; 36:729-734.

[24] D'Ambrosio E, Casa B, Bompani R, Scali G, Scali M. Glucosamine Sulfate: A Controlled Clinical Investigation in Arthrosis. Pharmacotherapeutica 1981; 2(8):504-508.

[25] Drovanti A, Bignamini AA, Rovati AL. Therapeutic Activity of Oral Glucosamine Sulfate in Osteoarthrosis: A Placebo-controlled Double-blind Investigation. *Clin Ther* 1998; 3:260-272.

[26] Dickenson, Annette, Who Uses Vitamin and Mineral Supplements?, http://www.crnusa.org/benpdfs/CRN011benefits_whovms.pdf

[27] Adebowale A, Cox D, et al. Analysis of Glucosamine and Chondroitin Sulfate Content in Marketed Products, http://www.ana-jana.org/reprints/EddingtonStudy.pdf

[28] Beal B. "Evaluation of Active Enzyme Activity in Six Oral Superoxide Dismutase Products." Paper presented at the 25th Annual Conference of the Veterinary Orthopedic Society, Snowmass, Colorado, 1998;65.

[29] Moore T. Messing with Mother Nature. *The Washingtonian* July 1999; 58-115.

[30] Li Y, Wang C, Zhu K, Feng RN, Sun CH., Effects of Multivitamin and Mineral Supplementation on Adiposity, Energy Expenditure and Lipid Profiles in Obese Chinese Women. Int J Obes (Lond). Feb 9, 2010.

[31] Ratey, John. *Spark - The Revolutionary New Science of Exercise and the Brain.* Little, Brown and Company; New York, NY 2008, p.236

[32] Cao H, Gerhold K, et al. Identification of a Lipokine, a Lipid Hormone Linking Adipose Tissue to Systemic Metabolism. Cell. 2008 Sep 19;134(6):933-44.

[33] Med Sci Sports Exerc. 1999 Nov;31(11 Suppl):S646-62. Effects of physical inactivity and obesity on morbidity and mortality: current evidence and research issues. Blair SN1, Brodney S.

[34] Flavell SW, Greenberg ME. Signaling mechanisms linking neuronal activity to gene expression and plasticity of the nervous system. *Annu Rev Neurosci.* 2008;31:563–590. doi:10.1146/annurev.neuro.31.060407.125631

[35] Panda, Satchin. The Circadian Code. Potter/Ten Speed/Harmony/Rodale. Kindle Edition.

[36] Circadian Misalignment in Mood Disturbances. Curr Psychiatry Rep. 2009 Dec;11(6):459-65.

[37] The Relation of Salivary Cortisol to Patterns of Performance on a Word List Learning Task in Healthy Older Adults. Psycho Nuero Endo. 2008 Oct;33(9):1293-6

[38] Circadian Stage-Dependent Inhibition of Human Breast Cancer Metabolism and Growth by the Nocturnal Melatonin Signal: Consequences of Its Disruption by Light at Night in Rats and Women. Integr Cancer Ther. 2009 Dec;8(4):347-53

[39] Circadian Clock and Vascular Disease. Hypertens Res. 2010 May 7.

[40] Melatonin-Insulin Interactions in Patients with Metabolic Syndrome. J Pineal Res. 2008 Jan;44(1):52-6.

[41] ibid

[42] https://www.ninds.nih.gov/Disorders/Patient-Caregiver-Education/Understanding-Sleep

[43] Panda, Satchin. The Circadian Code (p. 34). Potter/Ten Speed/Harmony/Rodale. Kindle Edition.

[44] Craig, Gary. http://www.selfgrowth.com/experts/gary_craig.html

[45] Walker, Scott. http://www.netmindbody.com/net

[46] https://www.becomingminimalist.com/un-busy/

[47] https://opinionator.blogs.nytimes.com/2012/06/30/the-busy-trap/

[48] Antenatal maternal anxiety and stress and the neurobehavioural development of the fetus and child: links and possible mechanisms. A review. Van den Bergh BR1, Mulder EJ, Mennes M, Glover V. Neurosci Biobehav Rev. 2005 Apr;29(2):237-58.

[49] Yoon MY, Yoon SS. Disruption of the Gut Ecosystem by Antibiotics. *Yonsei Med J.* 2017;59(1):4–12. doi:10.3349/ymj.2018.59.1.4

[50] Sontag SJ. The Medical Management of Reflux Esophagitis. Role of Antacids and Acid Inhibition. GastroenterolClin North Am. 1990 Sep;19(3):683-712.

[51] http://www.cdc.gov/ulcer/files/hpfacts.PDF

[52] Ching CK, Lam SK. Antacids. Indications and Limitations. Drugs. 1994 Feb;47(2):305-17.

[53] https://en.wikipedia.org/wiki/Milk-alkali_syndrome

[54] https://www.ncbi.nlm.nih.gov/pmc/articles/PMC4670772/

[55] Bicarbonate Concentration, Acid-Base Status, and Mortality in the Health, Aging, and Body Composition Study. Raphael KL, Murphy RA, et al. Clin J Am Soc Nephrol. 2016 Feb 5;11(2):308-16.

[57] https://teachmephysiology.com/gastrointestinal-system/stomach/acid-production/

[58] https://www.healthline.com/nutrition/the-alkaline-diet-myth#impact-of-food

[59] Nutritional disturbance in acid-base balance and osteoporosis: a hypothesis that disregards the essential homeostatic role of the kidney. Bonjour JP1. Br J Nutr. 2013 Oct;110(7):1168-77.

[60] Acid treatment of melanoma cells selects for invasive phenotypes. Moellering RE, Black KC, et al. Clin Exp Metastasis. 2008;25(4):411-25. Epub 2008 Feb 27.

[61] Phosphate Decreases Urine Calcium and Increases Calcium Balance: A Meta-analysis of the Osteoporosis Acid-Ash Diet Hypothesis. Fenton TR, Lyon AW, et al. Nutr J. 2009 Sep 15;8:41.

[62] Brownstein, David. Overcoming Arthritis. Medical Alternative Press, West Bloomfield MI, 2001. P. 154

[63] Batmanghelidj, F. Your Body's Many Cries for Water. http://www.watercure.com/

[64] Wright. Why Stomach Acid Is Good for You: Natural Relief from Heartburn, Indigestion, Reflux and GERD (p. 84). M. Evans & Company. Kindle Edition.

[65] Eidt S, Stolte M. The Significance of Helicobacter Pylori in Relation to Gastric Cancer and Lymphoma.Eur J GastroenterolHepatol. 1995 Apr;7(4):318-21.

[66] Cheon JH, Kim JH, et al. Helicobacter Pylori Eradication Therapy May Facilitate Gastric Ulcer Healing after Endoscopic Mucosal Resection: A Prospective Randomized Study. Helicobacter. 2008 Dec;13(6):564-71.

[67] Hunt, RH. *Helicobacter Pylori*: from Theory to Practice. Proceedings of a Symposium. Am J Med1996; 100 (5A) supplement.

[68] Kowalski M, Pawlik M, et al. Helicobacter Pylori Infection in Coronary Artery Disease. J PhysiolPharmacol. 2006 Sep;57Suppl 3:101-11.

[69] http://www.cdc.gov/ulcer/files/hpfacts.PDF

[70] Scarpignato C, Pelosini I, Di Mario F. Acid Suppression Therapy: Where Do We Go From Here? Dig Dis. 2006;24(1-2):11-46.

[71] Helicobacter pylori infection and chronic gastric acid hyposecretion. El-Omar EM[1], Oien K, et al. Gastroenterology. 1997 Jul;113(1):15-24.

[72] Beil W, Birkholz, Sewing KF. Effects of Flavonoids on Parietal Cell Acid Secretion, Gastric Mucosal Prostaglandin Production and Helicobacter Pylori Growth.ArzeneimForsch. 1995;45:697-700.

[73] Marle J, et al. Deglycrrhizinated Liquorice (DGL) and the Renewal of Rat Stomachepithelium. Eur J Pharm 1981;72:219.

[74] 11Kang Jy, et al. Effect of Colloidal Bismuth Subcitrate on Symptoms and Gastrichistology in Non-ulcer Dyspepsia. A Double Blind Placebo Controlled Study. Gut.1990;31: 476-480.

[75] https://www.ncbi.nlm.nih.gov/pmc/articles/PMC5772764/

[76] https://www.scientificamerican.com/article/gut-second-brain/

[77] The Roles of Inflammation, Nutrient Availability and the Commensal Microbiota in Enteric Pathogen Infection.
Stecher B. Microbiol Spectr. 2015 Jun;3(3). doi: 10.1128/microbiolspec.MBP-0008-2014.

[lxxviii] Gill RE, Hirst EL, Jones JK. Constitution of the Mucilage from the Bark of Ulmus Fulva (slippery elm mucilage); the Sugars Formed in the Hydrolysis of the Methylated Mucilage. J Chem Soc. 1946 Nov:1025-9.

[lxxix] Deters A, Zippel J, Hellenbrand N, Pappai D, Possemeyer C, Hensel A.
Aqueous Extracts and Polysaccharldes from Marshmallow roots (Althea
offi cinalis L.): cellular Internalisation and Stimulation of Cell Physiology of Human Epithelial Cells in Vitro. J Ethnopharmacol. 2010 Jan 8;127(1):62-9.

[lxxx] Marks IN, Boyd E. Mucosal Protective Agents in the Long-Term Management of Gastric Ulcer. Med J Aust. 1985 Feb 4;142(3):S23-5.

[lxxxi] Ekanem AP, Brisibe EA. Effects of Ethanol Extract of Artemisia Annua L. AgainstMonogenean Parasites of Heterobranchus Longifilis. Parasitol Res. 2010 Apr;106(5):1135-9.

[lxxxii] Belknap JK. Black Walnut Extract: An Inflammatory Model. Vet Clin North Am Equine Pract. 2010 Apr;26(1):95-101.

[lxxxiii] http://supremenutritionproducts.com/GoldenThreadSupreme/index.html

[84] Isaacs, Scott, Hormonal Balance, Understanding Hormones, Weight, and Your Metabolism. Bull Publishing, Boulder, Colorado. 2002. P.3

[85] https://www.nichd.nih.gov/health/topics/pcos

[86] Migraine. http://www.womenshealth.gov/faq/migraine.cfm#b

[87] ibid

[88] Edlow AG, Bartz D. Hormonal Contraceptive Options for Women with Headache: A Review of the Evidence. Rev Obstet Gynecol. 2010 Spring;3(2):55-65.

[89] https://www.rxlist.com/maxalt-side-effects-drug-center.htm

[90] Caspi A, Sugden K, et al. Influence of Life Stress on Depression: Moderation by a Polymorphism in the 5-HTT Gene. Science. 2003 Jul 18;301(5631):386-9.

[91] Schroeder M, Krebs MO, et al. Epigenetics and Depression: Current Challenges and New Therapeutic Options. Curr Opin Psychiatry. 2010 Jul 16.

[92] Szabo, Liz. The Number of Americans Taking Antidepressants Doubles. USA Today, 2009

[93]Ostrow, Nicole http://www.bloomberg.com/apps/news, nostrow1@bloomberg.net.

[94] Exercise Found Effective Against Depression. http://www.nytimes.com/2000/10/10/health/exercise-found-effective-against-depression.html

[95] Kubera M, Lin AH, Kenis G, Bosmans E, van Bockstaele D, Maes M. "Anti-Inflammatory Effects of Antidepressants Through Suppression of the Interferon-Gamma/Interleukin-10 Production Ratio." J Clin Psychopharmacol. 2001 Apr;21(2):199-206

[96] Maes M."The Immunoregulatory Effects of Antidepressants." Hum Psychopharmacol. 2001 Jan;16(1):95-103

[97] Ferguson JM. The Effects of Antidepressants on Sexual Functioning in Depressed Patients: A Review. J Clin Psychiatry. 2001;62 Suppl 3:22-34.

[98] Cougnard A, Verdoux H, Grolleau A, Moride Y, Begaud B, Tournier M. Impact of Antidepressants on the Risk of Suicide in Patients with Depression In Real-life Conditions: A Decision Analysis Model. Psychol Med. 2009 Aug;39(8):1307-15.

[99] Am J Public Health. 2004 May; 94(5): 746–747.

[100] American Autoimmune Related Diseases Association, Inc.

[101] Jacobson DL et al. Clin Immunol Immunopathol, 84: 223-243, 1997

[102] Pellicano R, Peyre S, et al. Updated Review on Helicobacter Pylori as a Potential Target for the Therapy of Ischemic Heart Disease (2006). Panminerva Med. 2006 Dec;48(4):241-6.

[103] Pellicano R, Parravicini PP, et al. Infection by Helicobacter Pylori and Acute Myocardial Infarction. Do Cytotoxic Strains Make a Difference? New Microbiol. 2002 Jul;25(3):315-21.

[104] Kharrazain, Datis. Why do I Still Have Thyroid Symptoms When my Lab Tests Are Normal? Morgan James Publishing. Garden City, New York; 2010

[105] Diamant M, Blaak EE, de Vos WM. Do Nutrient-Gut-Microbiota Interactions Play a Role in Human Obesity, Insulin Resistance and Type 2 Diabetes? Obes Rev. 2010 Aug 13.

[106] Neyrinck AM, Delzenne NM. Potential Interest of Gut Microbial Changes Induced by Non-Digestible Carbohydrates of Wheat in the Management of Obesity and Related Disorders. Curr Opin Clin Nutr Metab Care. 2010 Sep 4.

[107] Brownstein, David. Overcoming Arthritis. Medical Alternative Press, West Bloomfield MI, 2001. P. 13

[108] Subramanya D, Grivas PD. HPV and Cervical Cancer: Updates on an Established Relationship. Postgrad Med. 2008 Nov;120(4):7-13.

[109] Lawson JS. Do Viruses Cause Breast Cancer? Methods Mol Biol. 2009;471:421-38.

[110] Sauce D, Larsen M, et al. EBV-Associated Mononucleosis Leads to Long-Term Global Deficit in T-cell Responsiveness to IL-15. Blood. 2006 Jul 1;108(1):11-8.

[111] Fitch E, Harper E, et al. Pathophysiology of Psoriasis: Recent Advances on IL-23 and Th17 Cytokines. Curr Rheumatol Rep. 2007 Dec;9(6):461-7.

Made in the USA
Monee, IL
13 October 2023